# Yuck! Phlegm!

## HOW TO CLEAR YOUR PHLEGM USING IDEAS FROM CHINESE MEDICINE

JONATHAN CLOGSTOUN-WILLMOTT

Frame of Mind Publishing
Edinburgh, Scotland

# Contents

# Introduction to Phlegm, Catarrh, Snot ...

First, when you have read this book, may I ask you to review it?

This will help others decide if they might benefit from it. Please post your opinion on Amazon or anywhere else you think would reach prospective readers. Of course I hope you will write a positive or at least a constructive opinion!

However, if you have major reservations or criticisms, do let me know! Then I can improve the book for the next readers. Reach me through my website www.acupuncture-points.org, where on many pages there is a way to communicate with me.

*Why did I write this book?* And do I have much personal experience of phlegm?

Looking back I realise I suffered from phlegm from childhood. I was raised on a farm with Jersey cows, wonderful, docile and friendly animals that produced the richest creamy milk of all.

Our cows were grass-fed outside (except during snow) on what would now be regarded as organically-cultivated fields.

The milk I drank was neither pasteurised nor homogenised, just chilled. My mother used it to make yogurt and cream, ice-cream and occasionally cottage cheese.

I ate lots of it!

I frequently had ear-nose-throat problems. I had lots of phlegm. In fact I thought it normal. From time to time I had bad headaches, with phlegm blocking my sinuses, from which I recovered only with bed-rest, antibiotics and painkillers. I was also very spotty.

My father showed me how to clear my sinuses by sniffing up salty water.

It worked! – but only temporarily – because I then went and drank a mug of healthy, organically-grown, creamiest-of-all Jersey-cow milk!

Unfortunately it is now recognised even by doctors that milk tends to increase phlegm production.

Even now my body is inclined to produce phlegm, so I can honestly say that I have huge experience of it. Over the years I have groped my way to understanding it, and in this I have found Chinese medicine immensely informative and useful.

I have a website, written for my patients. I wrote a page about *phlegm*, and another about *phlegm after eating*. I was amazed at how popular they became, with visitors from all round the world, many thousands every month.

Reading other sites on phlegm I realised that many gave long lists of remedies but failed to explain which kinds of phlegm they were good for. So of course, what worked for one person would fail for another, with no-one the wiser.

So I have tried to distil quite a complicated subject into a useful book. Professional acupuncturists and practitioners of Chinese medicine will, I hope, accept that I have had to make simplifications of sometimes difficult conditions. But they may find some of the advice and herbal solutions useful for their patients: many of my patients helped me to formulate the advice here. Another reason for the book was because many asked how they could help themselves.

For phlegm, why is there such a range of possible treatments, and which one(s) work for you? (And yes, you can have more than one kind of phlegm at the same time!)

No two herbs or foods work exactly the same way. With

some, there are thousands of years of experience. With others, one must make some assumptions to decide how they work.

The same goes for medications prescribed by doctors which can confuse the underlying picture, removing important signs and adding others. For example,

- bronchodilators usually have a heating effect, reducing some signs of 'Cold' phlegm but adding some signs of 'Hot' phlegm;
- steroids eventually make you swell, increasing signs of 'Damp' and having overall a long-term weakening effect, even to the point of producing signs of 'Fatigue' phlegm;
- antibiotics are cold and damp, decreasing Hot phlegm but increasing signs of Damp phlegm and Cold phlegm.

These terms, Fatigue phlegm, Damp phlegm, Hot phlegm, Cold phlegm will become familiar by the end of the first chapter!

This book aims to help you to make sense of what kind of phlegm you have, what that probably means about your health and, once you understand the kind of phlegm you suffer from, what will often help you get rid of it.

Along the way, you'll pick up some of the ideas of Chinese medicine: very different from Western medicine and often making more sense or, at least, easier to put into effective practice without drugs.

Chapter 1 describes four different kinds of phlegm and one case of mucus and helps you decide which kind of phlegm you have. Knowing this is vital as each needs a different treatment to be successful.

Later you will read about the health history and mistakes made that probably led to each kind of phlegm.

From that alone you may see how to get yourself better.

Chapters 3 to 7 cover underlying patterns of health and disease that often lead to phlegm production. These are the root causes of phlegm. If you don't address them your phlegm will return, as I have learned the hard way. These chapters contain the most theory, but once you understand them, solutions become obvious.

Chapter 9 lists many of the phlegm solutions proposed in books or on the internet and begins to analyse them to see how they may be useful to you.

Chapters 10 – 14 puts everything together for five different kinds of phlegm, giving you clear suggestions to help yourself.

Chapter 15 is a short chapter describing or listing how other kinds of phlegm upset your health, some seriously.

Because some of the ideas in Chinese medicine take a bit of explanation, I have mostly put links to them as they are introduced. These links go to my website. Because I know readers will tend to skip to the chapters that interest them, these links are repeated frequently throughout the text.

This repetition is intentional and will irk readers who dislike repetition, but I think they make reading the book easier if it is read using a computer, tablet, smart-phone, Kindle or similar. To include full explanations in the text would make the book too long.

I expect to revise and improve the book from time to time.
Jonathan Clogstoun-Willmott
June 2017

# Chapter 1 What Kind of Phlegm do you have?

Before going further, please note that this book is about *ongoing* phlegm, *chronic* phlegm which you have had for some time, long past any acute illness that brought it on, such as a cold or worse.

In other words, this book is **not** about the phlegm you have *during* a cold or other intense, acute illness. *This book is about phlegm that hangs around afterwards, slowing you down for days, months or years, or always returns for ages after an acute illness.*

So, what kind of phlegm do you have?

Overcome your revulsion and have a good look at it! Spit some out onto white paper or a white handkerchief.

Is your **phlegm – ? –**

- watery ie colourless
- runny
- white
- brown
- yellow

- green
- thick
- made up of little pellets
- viscid and/or stringy
- containing blood, ie bloody

## Tongue Body

Now have a look at your tongue! Stick it out and consider it. Is the **body** of your tongue (as opposed to the surface *coating*) – ?
–

- pale
- red
- purple
- wet or dry
- swollen, or swollen in places
- teeth-marked along the edges
- with a crease down the middle

## Tongue Coating

Then what about the surface **coating**?

- absent
- white
- brown
- yellow or green
- greasy or sticky

- colourless
- peeled off in patches

### Your Pulse – your heartbeat

Now count your pulse per minute:

- Under 55: slow
- Between 65 and 75: normal
- Over 85: fast

Right! Already you have acquired a whole pile of information that you can use in diagnosing what kind of phlegm you have. Knowing that will help you understand how to get rid of it.

Although there are many more kinds of phlegm explained in Chinese medicine, I've reduced them to five types. If your type of phlegm is not explained here, I apologise, but this book aims to help most – probably 80% – kinds of 'substantial' phlegm – 'substantial' meaning you can spit it out and touch it, should you wish to! The other 20% needs careful evaluation, diagnosis and treatment from a professional practitioner with knowledge of Chinese medicine's theory.

(What about *'non-substantial' phlegm,* I hear you ask? That can be more serious, depending on ... well, see chapter 15. Anyway, non-substantial phlegm cannot be spat out or touched.)

## HOW TO USE THE INFORMATION YOU'VE GATHERED

### Colour of your phlegm

As you realise, the colour of your phlegm may range between colourless to white then green via yellow. What do these colours mean?

## Colourless ie watery

**Colourless** phlegm is rather like mucus but thicker. (Mucus is the normal fluid that keeps your mucus membranes moist, rather like saliva.) If colourless, and more so if it is also watery, your phlegm has not had enough heat on it to thicken or colour it. So it is more likely to be from either *fatigue*, or from *damp* or from *cold*.

- *Fatigue* occurs as you get tired! This happens towards the evening after a day's work, or when, having worked hard for many months you realise you need a holiday; or after a severe debilitating illness, including after a respiratory illness even if not 'serious'. For more on fatigue see http://www.acupuncture-points.org/qi.html and http://www.acupuncture-points.org/excess-or-deficient.html. In the theory of Chinese medicine, what I call 'fatigue phlegm' is not actually phlegm at all, but profuse mucus. I include it here because it is not uncommon and you can usually do something about it yourself.

- *Damp* occurs in damp places, and is often a cause of many kinds of illness. Damp can occur in hot places too, such as during the monsoon season, and of course in cold countries where it often rains. 'Damp phlegm' is usually white, profuse in quantity and with little smell or taste. However, having said that, most Damp phlegm comes from what and how you eat. For more on Damp see http://www.acupuncture-points.org/damp.html

- *Cold* invades you from outside your body, from the weather, from having too much cold food or drink, or from exposure to cold conditions or environments, such as working in a freezing environment, or in a cold marketplace early in the morning, or by sitting on something cold for too long. Read more about cold at http://www.acupuncture-points.org/

cold.html. 'Cold phlegm' is usually white and watery but can be thicker and more glutinous, because the Cold has thickened it, as soup thickens when cold.

Just as urine is usually darker first thing in the morning,  so the colour of your phlegm becomes darker the longer it remains in your body. (By the way, if you take nutritional supplements, or vitamin B complex, or some foods such as beetroot, your urine will temporarily darken.)

So phlegm expectorated first thing in the morning may be slightly coloured, perhaps a little yellow, but almost colourless later in the day. This could still be fatigue phlegm, damp phlegm or cold phlegm.

## Runny phlegm

Usually comes from Fatigue or Damp, sometimes from Cold, but phlegm from Cold is often thicker. Other factors would help you decide.

## White phlegm

Usually means Cold or Damp are your problems. If thick *and* white, can sometimes mean Heat phlegm. Other factors would help you decide.

## Brown phlegm

Usually means means old Heat, unless you have just eaten or drunk something coloured. Old Heat could come from a history of tobacco smoking, for example.

## Yellow or green phlegm?

Just as some chemicals change colour when heated, so your phlegm becomes more yellow, even green, as your body heats it. This **yellow or green is the colour of Hot phlegm**. (Well, nearly always! Watery or white phlegm *could* also arise from Heat, but these are rare and too complicated for now.)

As phlegm is heated, other changes occur. The heat also dries and thickens it, so that usually yellow or green phlegm is less runny than Fatigue phlegm, Damp phlegm or Cold phlegm.

If your phlegm is both a strong yellow and very runny, and assuming you haven't eaten anything to colour it, it would probably be diagnosed as being due to both Heat *and* Damp. For confirmation you would look at other features, such as the shape of your tongue and its coating.

## Thick phlegm

Thick phlegm can look globular, lumpy or heavy. This takes time or intensity to form, and time usually means either you have Cold or Heat in your system. Cold slows and congeals fluids; Heat dries and condenses them.

You decide whether Cold or Heat is the cause mainly from the colour of the phlegm, although other factors play an important part too, as you'll understand as you read on. Cold phlegm tends to be white or sometimes colourless, Hot phlegm is more coloured, either yellow or green or dark.

Colour intensity means that your symptoms, perhaps those of a recent illness, e.g. a cold, have been intense or strong.

## Phlegm made of pellets

Pellets are little bits of phlegm, discrete in size, and may appear in small quantities, often in thicker phlegm. Here your body has taken thick phlegm and solidified it. As with thick phlegm, you can usually tell the cause from the colour: white pellets are from Cold, yellow pellets are from Heat.

That they are pellets suggests they come from deeper within your lungs. That you can expectorate them is good because it shows your body has enough energy to do so. On the other hand, pellets in your lungs will have reduced your breathing ability and energy, probably for some time – not so good.

### Viscid, stringy phlegm

Like pellets, viscid phlegm takes longer to form. It suggests that you have had phlegm in your system for some time or very intensely. Its colour tells you whether due to Cold or Heat. Usually Cold phlegm is white, Hot phlegm is yellow or green.

### Bloody phlegm

Blood in your phlegm nearly always means Heat but can occasionally mean Fatigue.

In either case, **before embarking on suggestions made in this book** *I urge you to seek medical advice*.

### Your tongue

Tongue diagnosis is based on over 1000 years experience in Chinese medicine and takes years to master, although one can learn the basics quite fast. The following is only a brief summary of this important subject but can help you decide which kind of phlegm problem you have.

## Tongue Body

### *Pale tongue*

A pale tongue suggests *Blood deficiency* (http://www.acupuncture-points.org/blood.html), meaning that your body is failing either to produce or manufacture enough blood, or to move it to where it is needed. Blood deficient tongues are less moist than you might expect, because Blood provides the moisture and Blood deficiency means less of it.

So, if it is also wet, a pale tongue can also mean *deficiency of warming-moving* energy (ie energy of a *'yang'* nature – for more on yang and yin, see http://www.acupuncture-points.org/yin-and-yang.html) in your body. Yang deficiency is a common cause of phlegm, especially damp phlegm and cold phlegm. You can usually do something about it yourself.

### *Red tongue*

A healthy tongue is pink: a red tongue is, well, redder!

Extra redness means *Heat (*http://www.acupuncture-points.org/Heat.html).

However, now it gets complicated because assuming the tongue has a solid coating, that heat comes from what is called *Full* heat. If the coating is absent or partial the redness probably means *Empty* heat.

*Full* heat usually means a recent infection or fever.

*Empty* heat means the metabolic processes of the body are producing heat without there being a recent infection or fever. Often this is caused by Yin deficiency, a condition not recognised in Western medicine but important in Chinese medicine. See more at http://www.acupuncture-points.org/yin-deficiency.html

*Purple or dark*

A purple tongue has an important meaning – *Blood Stasis*. This syndrome is more common in older people and can lead on to many potentially serious conditions. Read more at http://www.acupuncture-points.org/blood-stasis.html.

From the point of view of this book, Blood stasis tends to make phlegm worse (and vice versa) but explaining why takes us away from the main purpose of the book which is to explain and help you manage and clear the common forms of phlegm.

*Wet or Dry*

In health, a tongue is moist, not dry and not very wet.

Too dry and it suggests *heat* or a *lack of moisture* in the system, especially in your digestion and Stomach.

Very wet suggests *Yang deficiency* (http://www.acupuncture-points.org/yang-deficiency.html) and probably *Damp* http://www.acupuncture-points.org/damp.html.

*Swollen*

With just about all the main forms of phlegm, the body of the tongue is swollen i.e. bigger than usual. However, swelling doesn't always mean phlegm: it could be due to fluid accumulation somewhere which might be oedema, for example or Damp.

*Where* your tongue is swollen says a lot about your problem.

- Towards but just behind the tip of your tongue: phlegm is mainly resident in your lungs, and/or your Lungs' ability to disperse phlegm is compromised – see chapter 5.

- In the middle of the tongue: phlegm comes from weak

digestion or the wrong diet – what in Chinese medicine is called your Spleen energy – see chapters 3 & 4.

- On the sides of the tongue (which may show what look like tooth-marks) suggests a history either of Qi-stagnation, which may be because of postural or stress problems – see chapter 7: or fatigue, chapters 3,4 and 10. See also next paragraph on Tooth-marks.

*Tooth-marks*

Tooth-marks on the sides of your tongue usually mean what is called 'Spleen deficiency'. This can mean:

- Tiredness and fatigue, your body unable to move blood around to nourish itself
- Stress, causing what is called 'Qi Stagnation' (for instance http://www.acupuncture-points.org/liver-qi-stagnation.html) has tightened up your 'Liver' (http://www.acupuncture-points.org/liver-functions.html) making it 'squeeze' your Spleen!
- A swollen tongue, swollen perhaps from Damp or Phlegm, which in themselves point to a weakened Spleen
- Nothing at all – your tongue may be normal.
- Besides reading chapters 3 & 4, for more on your Spleen see http://www.acupuncture-points.org/spleen.html

*Centre crease*

A small crease along the mid-line of the tongue may mean little, but if accentuated it means Spleen and Stomach problems, either now, or eventually.

This is normally deficiency of Stomach 'yin', meaning of

Stomach fluids, such as of hydrochloric acid or of mucus that prevents the acid from destroying the lining of the stomach. Lack of these fluids means you don't digest food so well and (see chapter 4) a poor digestion easily leads to phlegm.

Creases elsewhere, short or long, sometimes mean little. More often they suggest either yin deficiency (http://www.acupuncture-points.org/yin-deficiency.html), a past history of fevers (possibly long-past, as in childhood), or an inherited susceptibility to disease.

## Tongue Coating

**No coating, i.e. coating absent:** your Stomach lacks normal fluids, including acid and mucus protecting its lining. This indicates that your stomach does not have enough wherewithal to digest food: not enough Stomach 'Qi' as it is called.

During good treatment the tongue coating should regenerate to the point where it becomes normal i.e. thin and white.

As you grow older, your digestion tends to become less efficient and so older people are those who more commonly lack tongue coating.

A **colourless** coating means a deficiency of Stomach Yang energy. A **thin white** coating is normal.

A **thick** coating, meaning you cannot see the tongue's body through it, suggests what is called a 'pathogenic factor' in your body. A pathogenic factor invades your body, causing you to get ill, e.g. from a virus or bacteria such as a cold or measles. For more on what I mean by a pathogenic factor, see http://www.acupuncture-points.org/external-causes-of-disease.html.

- If **thick** and **white** this usually means Cold. That means your body has reacted to the invader with a 'cold' reaction. Normally this makes you feel cold.

- If **thick** and **yellow or green**, it means Heat. That means your body has reacted to the invader with a 'hot' reaction. Normally this makes you feel hot.

A **greasy, sticky** coating usually means Damp (http://www.acupuncture-points.org/damp.html) or Phlegm.

A **peeled** tongue: with a peeled tongue, which looks as if patches of its coating have been peeled off, leaving 'raw' tongue body underneath, the usual cause is strong medication, often antibiotics. This reflects the devastating effect the medication has had on your gastro-intestinal tract, denuding it of beneficial flora and fluids. (Other medicines have other effects. For example steroids often make the tongue swell, indicating damp or phlegm in your system, which may be reflected in your face, which looks bright, shiny and slightly puffed up.)

For more on tongue diagnosis, see http://www.acupuncture-points.org/tongue-diagnosis.html

Summarising, you could say that a tongue which is

- swollen with either a colourless or slightly white coating, sticky or greasy, suggests Damp phlegm

- swollen with a wet, white coating suggests Cold Phlegm

- swollen with a yellow coating means Hot phlegm

- swollen and dry or with a central crease containing phlegm, is probably Dry phlegm

- no swelling, but wet and with a thin white or transparent coating, possibly with indentations on the sides, means Fatigue phlegm.

## What about your pulse?

This is much simpler! Basically (of course there are exceptions but, sticking to phlegm ...)

• A slow pulse means Cold
• A fast pulse means Heat

The pulse for Damp phlegm may be normal in speed.

A slow pulse is often found in people who have at some time in their lives trained physically very intensively, meaning they are or were athletes or sporty. Western medicine sees no problem in this, indeed tends to applaud it.

Chinese medicine is not so happy about a slow pulse, which suggests that your body has not been able to maintain proper pulse speed for some reason, meaning a lack of energy (more accurately, a lack of Qi, not quite the same thing – http://www.acupuncture-points.org/qi.html) or of yang (http://www.acupuncture-points.org/yang-deficiency.html), neither of which is conducive to good health. Qi and Yang deficiencies make you more susceptible to disease respectively (in Western terms) from lowered vitality and inefficient metabolic reactivity.

A trained acupuncturist can read far more from your pulse, and may take many minutes to do it! Also, during treatment, many acupuncturists often refer back to your pulse to see what difference their treatment is making. Often the right treatment changes your pulse quality within seconds, whereas changes on the tongue take far longer, often hours or days.

For more on your pulse and what can be diagnosed from it, read http://www.acupuncture-points.org/pulse-diagnosis.html

## DIAGNOSING YOUR PHLEGM!

So, at last you come to diagnosing your phlegm.

As you will read in chapter 15, there are many kinds of phlegm, but the ones we are interested in are all what is called 'substantial' phlegm, meaning the *stuff that you can hawk or cough up and spit out*.

In other words *you can touch it*.

Note: items below in bold are more obvious and important. Other items listed become more likely the longer you have had your condition.

You will notice that how your phlegm is diagnosed depends not just on what the phlegm looks like but on other factors.

This is important because otherwise you might think Damp phlegm was identical to Cold phlegm – but you could easily have both together!

## 1. FATIGUE PHLEGM

Fatigue phlegm is not actually phlegm, but extra mucus. Confusingly, it can arise with any of the other kinds of phlegm.

- **Lots of mucus** – not the same as phlegm!
- Nose runs easily
- Eyes water easily in bright light or a breeze, more so if it's cold
- Mouth may dribble, for example during sleep
- You urinate more easily or more often than usual
- **Shortness of breath**
- Often a slight cough brings up thin, watery stuff.
- Facial oedema

- Nausea – but this is rare. If you bring up stomach fluids they are runny and lack strong acid taste.
- **Loss of voice**, or voice is weaker than usual
- Possible perspiration when you would not expect it
- You feel tired – as you might feel at the end of a long day's work, or when you really need a holiday
- Tongue: pale
- Tongue body; not swollen, may or may not have a crease down the middle, but if so, is usually not a deep crease
- Tongue body may have indentations like teeth-marks on the sides, which are even more likely if you have been stressed. Teeth-marks can indicate stress but also fatigue.
- Signs of Fatigue phlegm sometimes occur in people who have been using steroids for a long time
- Can combine with other forms of phlegm, such as Damp phlegm, Cold phlegm.
- Very occasionally it combines with Dry phlegm, which is very confusing and better treated by a professional.
- See chapters 3, 4, 5, 6, 7 and 10.

## 2. DAMP PHLEGM

'Damp' suggests wetness so with damp-phlegm you get

- **copious quantities of the stuff, easy to expectorate**
- **phlegm is white or colourless, often runny**
- Very occasionally, Damp phlegm is 'jade-green' in colour.
- **phlegm is often sticky**
- **lack of thirst; or dry mouth but no desire to drink**

- **fullness or heaviness in chest and upper abdomen (ie in your chest and epigastrium)**
- can feel lumps in the chest
- **cough sounds thick and full of phlegm**
- **nausea, poor appetite**, possibly even at the sight of greasy or very rich or sweet food; nausea **often worse on waking in the morning**
- desires sweet food and drinks
- **tongue body is swollen with a crease down the middle**
- excess salivation
- lethargy or tendency to feel more sleepy than usual
- tendency to worry, to overthink, which may prevent sleep, can be depressed
- poor concentration
- forgetful
- headache
- head feels full and stuffy
- vertigo
- muscles and joints may be stiff
- heaviness and lethargy, which are often worse in the early morning, before or as you get moving. After you get moving, the heaviness and lethargy ease somewhat
- **after eating, your phlegm may be more profuse,** and you need to clear your throat before speaking
- after eating you feel heavier and less able to think for a while, as if too full: possibly you need to loosen your clothing
- **tongue coating is sticky and either colourless or a little white, often greasy**

- tongue body may be flabby
- pulse is usually neither fast nor slow but if the condition is bad, it may be a little slower than normal. Its 'quality' to an acupuncturist would be 'slippery', possibly 'floating'.
- **You feel worse in wet or damp rooms, weather conditions, environments or climates**
- If you have had these symptoms for years, your body may easily gain weight
- In long-term conditions of damp-phlegm, the complexion may become dull or even blackish
- If you have had this for a long time, you may look heavy, fatigued, overweight, with the tendency to overeat whenever your appetite returns
- you probably have a background of not eating the right foods for good health
- Signs of Damp phlegm sometimes occur in people who have used antibiotics or steroids for a long time
- Can easily combine with Cold phlegm or Fatigue phlegm, less frequently with Hot phlegm.
- See chapters 3, 4, 5, 6, 7 and 11.

## 3. COLD PHLEGM

'Cold' suggests that you may be cold, or that your body lacks enough heat to respond to its problems, and that you prefer warmth.

- **Your phlegm is usually clear, thin and stringy but can be white or watery, even thick and glutinous,** depending on how long or intensively you have had the condition
- **Your chest feels heavy and full: 'stuffy'**

- **Your arms and legs feel cold**
- **Your arms and legs feel heavy**
- **You get excess salivation**
- Your cough is worse (ie more frequent) in cold conditions or cold air, winter, night, or if undressing in a cool room
- Nausea
- Your abdomen feels distended and can feel cold
- Head feels heavy and you feel 'slow', worse in the morning
- **Tongue body is pale and swollen; may have a crease down the middle**
- **Desire to lie still and keep warm**
- Tendency to fluid retention i.e. oedema, worse in your lower body or legs, ankles or feet
- Urination may be scanty or difficult
- Cold ache in your low back and legs, knees
- Stools are loose and may contain little bits of undigested food (technical name for this is 'lienteric')
- Face is pale
- **Tongue coating is wet and white, can look greasy or slippery**
- Tongue body is pale, swollen, flabby
- **Pulse is slow –** usually, and to an acupuncturist it would feel 'slippery', possibly slightly 'tight' or 'wiry', often 'deep'
- **You feel worse in cold rooms, weather conditions, environments or climates**
- You may also feel worse in overcast or damp conditions
- You feel better in warm weather, summer or a dry autumn

- **You like warmth on your chest and abdomen**
- You may be elderly
- You may be someone who lifted weights or heavy objects too much in the past, or – if male, had too much ejaculatory sex for your kind of constitution
- Signs of Cold phlegm sometimes occur in people who have used antibiotics for while, or frequently
- Can combine with Damp phlegm and Fatigue phlegm. Treat the Cold phlegm as first priority.
- See chapters 3, 4, 5, 6, 7 and 12.

## 4. HOT PHLEGM

'Hot' suggests a past fever but still a feeling of heat.

- **Phlegm is thick, yellow or green, and sticky**; *sometimes* is thick and white, possibly globular
- Cough is more frequent in heat, warm air or a warm room
- If Heat is strong, **phlegm is hard to expectorate** or cough up as it has become too thick and solid, almost rubbery
- Chest feels oppressed, can be an effort to breathe
- Nausea
- **Mouth feels dry or has a sticky sensation**
- **Thirst, usually for frequent cool fluids, unless also Damp-phlegm, when often thirstless**
- **Face is red**
- **Head can feel distended, swollen**
- May tend to be feverish, depending on how strong the Heat
- Ears are more sensitive to noise

- **Restlessness,** anxiety, even palpitations
- Skin is often greasy or moist: face can look as if oiled
- **Prefers cool air**
- Heavy feeling is worse in the morning
- Urination is scanty, may be sore to urinate; urine is darker than normal
- Constipation
- Body odour is strong
- **Tongue body is swollen** and often red in colour; almost certainly **has a crease down the middle**
- The tongue crease may have dry or sticky yellow phlegm inside it
- **Tongue coating is often yellow,** thick and **sticky or greasy;** sometimes peeled off in patches
- Taste may be bitter or sticky
- **Pulse is faster than usual**; to an acupuncturist it might feel 'slippery', 'thready' or 'thin', even 'wiry'; 'surging'
- **You feel worse in warm or hot rooms, 'muggy' weather conditions, environments or climates**
- You feel worse in noisy conditions
- **You feel a little better in cool conditions**
- With this condition you may snore when normally you don't, or snore more if normally you do!
- Some medications such as broncho-dilators can increase Heat in users, who get thirstier or drier (eg throat or skin) than they otherwise might be, or become more restless or get palpitations, with thicker, whiter phlegm than they would have without medication. Of course, if they had pre-existing

Hot phlegm, broncho-dilators may worsen some of the Heat symptoms, even if they make the chest feel less oppressed and breathing easier.

- Hot phlegm can combine with Dry phlegm, see below. Very occasionally it combines with Fatigue phlegm, in which case treat it first as Hot phlegm.

- See chapters 3, 4, 5, 6, 7 and 13.

## 5. DRY PHLEGM

'Dry' means that phlegm has dried and is very hard to shift.

- **Dry cough**, worse in hot or dry air, warm rooms, in hot streams of air such as from a fan heater
- **Phlegm is yellow or yellow-white, powdery or pellety or stringy, sticky and stretchy (viscid): thread-like globules: hard to cough up or expectorate**
- **Chest feels oppressed, heavy, tight, constrained: may have wheezing**
- **Inside nose feels dry**
- **Throat feels dry or with small amounts of phlegm**
- **Mouth feels dry**
- Phlegm brought up may contain blood
- Shortness of breath
- Stools are dry and hard to 'move'
- Urine is scanty and dark
- Skin is dry
- Fever is possible
- If yin deficiency is present there will be a sensation of heat in

the afternoon, possibly with noises in the ears, sweating at night, back-pain, restlessness and anxiety, scanty urine, frequent small thirst, dry skin and hair. Yin deficiency is a big subject, (see http://www.acupuncture-points.org/yin-deficiency.html) and occurs more as people age, and Dry phlegm does tend to occur more in the aged

- Head feels heavy or muzzy

- Mild dizziness

- Complexion is dry and pasty coloured

- **Tongue body is swollen, usually with a crease down the middle. The crease often contains phlegm.**

- Tongue coating is white, thin and dry, may be sticky, sometimes yellow. Described sometimes as 'sticky lacquer'.

- Tongue body colour: tip may be red.

- Pulse may fast if there is also ongoing Heat, and to an acupuncturist would feel 'slippery'.

- This tends to occur when you have been subjected to a very dry environment in the past, or as you age, with a history of Hot phlegm or as yin deficiency develops.

- Some medications such as broncho-dilators can increase Dryness in users, who get thirstier or drier (eg throat or skin) than they otherwise might be, or become more restless or get palpitations, with thicker, whiter phlegm than they might have. If they had pre-existing Hot phlegm, broncho-dilators may worsen some of the symptoms, even if the chest feels less oppressed and breathing easier.

- Can combine with Hot phlegm, very occasionally with Fatigue phlegm.  If so seek advice as to which to treat first.

- See chapters 3, 4, 5, 6, 7 and 14.

OK! You should be able to decide at least between dry or hot phlegm on the one hand and cold or damp phlegm on the other. But I admit that distinguishing the different types takes practice, and that you can easily have combinations, though you would not normally have both *hot* phlegm *and cold* phlegm at the same time. (But it *could* seem like it! In which case let someone else, preferably experienced, help you decide.)

Now you need to know about how these different forms of phlegm come into existence, what you have been doing to acquire your kind of phlegm and, importantly, why you still have it – why it has become chronic.

This 'maintaining' or root cause is the chief factor to understand if you really want to clear your phlegm, long-term.

The next six chapters explain this.

# Chapter 2 - How Chinese Medicine goes about explaining Snot!

I visited China for 6 months starting in the autumn of 1982. Part of the time I worked in a hospital clinic specialising in acupuncture, part of the time I attended lectures, and the rest of the time, I travelled or was taken around.

Beijing was grey with dust from the Mongolian plains and from the huge building works in progress. Many people had nasal and phlegm problems. Nanjing, where I did the course, had less Mongolian dust, but plenty of building works. More importantly, what people ate was often greasy, fatty and sweet. The local authority was so vexed by the population's bad habits that it put spittoons in the streets, with phlegm wardens to arrest anyone seen spitting elsewhere.

So we may think we have phlegm problems, but the Chinese have them just as badly! This in spite of 2500 years of a medicine now increasingly respected and used worldwide. However, the way Chinese medicine was used at that time in China was more practical than educational: if a patient sought treatment he or she would be advised what to eat and given treatment for the problem, but there was no obvious teaching or long-term support or encouragement.

However, older generations had knowledge handed down through the generations. Grandparents who had survived both the Chinese civil war from 1927 to 1950 and the invasion by and war with Japan 1937-46 brought with them what we might describe as 'old wives' tales', or kitchen medicine.

However, that kitchen medicine had long since evolved into the modern miracle that is Chinese medicine, especially Chinese herbal medicine. But when I worked in Nanjing 1982-83, many older people would walk into the clinic and tell us, using the terminology of Chinese medicine, what they thought their problem was. (For instance, an elderly woman with cystitis told us she thought she had 'Cold in her Kidneys': she was right! One treatment using warmth via moxibustion (http://www.acupuncture-points.org/moxibustion.html) on some needles cured it. However, don't assume all cystitis is Cold in the Kidneys!)

The problem for Westerners is that, unlike Western medicine, which has a medicine for everything, including phlegm, Chinese herbs and treatments must be individualised: each person's condition must be carefully diagnosed.

Once the correct diagnosis is made, appropriate treatment follows, including advice about what to do to help yourself. So no generalised tonics can be taken safely, because what helps one diagnosis might worsen another.

The advantage is that with the correct diagnosis and treatment, the underlying problem which allowed the phlegm to collect is itself corrected. That makes the phlegm less likely to recur. Contrast that with Western medicine, where the OTC 'over the counter' drug may suppress the phlegm for a while only, but it is not in the interests of the pharmaceutical industry to advise how to avoid it.

So what has 2500 years of Chinese medicine, including their 'kitchen' medicine, have to say about phlegm?

In Chinese medicine, phlegm is a big subject. That's good news for you: it means they've probably got an answer for most of your problems! The bad news is that some 'phlegm' diseases are difficult to cure without professional treatment – see chapter 15.

On the other hand, there are many situations where Chinese medicine can quickly cure phlegm, and give you good advice about how to help yourself without professional treatment.

*The next four chapters explain how your body keeps phlegm at bay, and what happens when this goes wrong.*

# Chapter 3 - Your 'Spleen': thoughts, feelings and habits

Your spleen **organ** lies under your lower left ribs, beside and partly behind your stomach. It cleans your blood, recycles old red blood cells and helps with your immunity.

However, by your 'Spleen', Chinese medicine means rather more. It could be said to include all the functions of your spleen organ, but it goes much further. You could say that your 'Spleen' (capital S) is Cook, Cleaner and Maintenance or Plumber, though even that hardly does it justice.

It is more like a general housekeeper.

- As Cook, it turns what you eat into healthy blood and energy
- As Cleaner, it clears debris and recycles rubbish, bringing fresh supplies to all parts
- As Maintenance and Plumber, it repairs tissue

What happens when the Spleen fails?

- You run out of energy and may become anaemic
- Your body gets ill more easily

- Your skin loses it healthy 'bloom'
- Garbage collects! What does garbage look like? Phlegm!

However, that's not the end of the story because other factors make phlegm –

- thinner, more like water
- thicker, like cream
- green
- yellow
- white
- red
- drier, into lumps, or strings, or even powder

and make phlegm appear in different places, in your –

- nose
- throat
- lungs
- mouth (and if in your mouth, *where* it occurs can make a big difference to understanding what is going on)
- stools
- skin, near the surface, such as in abscesses
- skin, deeper, such as fatty nodules
- ears, like wax

What makes your Spleen 'fail'?
    This has been the subject of careful observation and thought for over 2500 years.
    It turns out that as far as the Spleen goes, we can *ourselves*

often do something about reducing or eliminating phlegm. This is because we can learn how to eat the right food and not the wrong stuff. *How* we eat and *what* we eat are two separate and important issues.

Emotions also play a huge part in our health and digestion, far more than you may suspect! By living with more equanimity you can reduce the effects on your health and, specially on your Spleen, of unruly thoughts and feelings.

The rest of this chapter deals with the emotional and mental issues. The next chapter – 4 – deals with food issues and the environment and how these affect your Spleen.

## EMOTIONS

You may think your emotions have nothing to do with your phlegm. You are wrong! True, emotions don't often produce phlegm immediately, unlike some foods or food combinations in susceptible individuals – see next chapter.

But emotions can be more insidious, undermining our equanimity. Chinese thought considers that your Spleen works best when calm and unhurried. How you think has a huge affect on your Spleen's efficiency.

### The Plumber

Like an experienced plumber or handyman, able to mend almost any household problem, your Spleen works best when allowed to get on with the job. If the plumber is assailed by your (or his) tantrums, panics or worries, he won't be able to do the work: either it won't get done, or it will take longer.

If the work is completed in a rush, it may break down again. Let your plumber get on with it: and don't talk to him too much, either! That's the equivalent of over-thinking; taking time you are paying for that stops him from getting on with the job.

For any householder dependent on a good plumber, the last thing you want is that he suddenly stops work on your boiler to answer an emergency call somewhere else. You want him to stay with you until the work is completed.

In the same way, you can disturb the smooth functioning of your Spleen and your digestion by concentrating on more than one thing at a time. If you try to do too many things at once, using your mind like a search-light, first on this then on that then the other, you will be unsettled.

Signs that your Spleen is unsettled and that your body is trying to compensate, to keep it on track, are if you habitually chew something, drink (eg tea) or bite or pick your lips or fingers, grind your teeth or suck your teeth. Each of these stimulates your mouth and throat, (even picking at your fingers) which in Chinese medicine relate to the Stomach and Spleen one way or another. The same goes for smoking a cigarette or vape, because your lips hold them – but smoke also stimulates your Lungs, of which see chapter 5.

The Stomach descends food: or it should, otherwise you feel nausea and the food comes up again! By stimulating your lips, teeth, tongue, oral cavity and throat, you are prodding your Stomach and Spleen to descend 'energy' (if you have nothing in your mouth) or food, if you are chewing something. That helps keep you centred and relaxed, able to concentrate on your work.

This is, we all realise (don't we?), the equivalent as a baby of sucking our fingers or a dummy-pacifier. It helps to calm us down. Apparently we start sucking our fingers in the womb! These ancient, deep-seated habits are hard to change.

There are other ways of doing this, including picking our fingers, commonly the thumb and forefinger – and in Chinese medicine there's even a reason for why we choose these fingers rather than the others. (I was different! Apparently I sucked my middle and ring fingers, no doubt explaining – if I could understand it – where my life went wrong!)

Your thumb relates to your lungs and your forefinger to your intestines, mainly your large intestine but also your stomach, because the acupuncture channels of those names start on those fingers. Your Lungs have a major connection with your Stomach and Spleen energies, so by sucking your thumb your are pacifying both your Lungs and your Spleen and Stomach.

(By the way, there's a reason why sometimes organs are spelled with a small letter and sometimes with a Capital letter. For example, lungs and Lungs. The small letter (lungs) means the organ. The Capital letter (Lungs) means the energy and sphere of application, including the organ in question, in this case of the Lungs. And sometimes, to confuse you, it hasn't been corrected in the editing.)

Guess which way your Lungs send energy (in Chinese medicine)? Down!

There's a reason for this: stimulating your mouth stimulates your Stomach energy to 'descend', making you swallow more often or, in the case of smoking, to inhale more. The descending functions of the Lungs or Stomach temporarily stimulate your Spleen energy to work better. That helps you stay focused. So that's good.

But of course there are plenty of people who don't pick their lips, don't chew gum, don't suck their teeth or smoke and so on. What about them? Well, they get tense in other ways and that causes them a host of problems which (here's an unashamed plug for it) I wrote a book about: http://www.acupuncture-points.org/qi-stagnation.html.

The downside is that you get fat or, if you smoke, you damage your lungs. Too many cups of tea or coffee also make you pee more, further disturbing your working patterns.

So try to do one thing at a time. Keep calm. Do it for a reasonable period of time, then switch to another job.

- Avoid answering the phone too often. Put your phone on voicemail or get someone else to respond to calls and ask them to make a list of people you must ring.
- If your work is manual, explain to supervisors the nonsense of trying to do two different jobs at once, or being asked to undertake other activities when the first is incomplete
- If at your desk, complete one job, then move to the next.
- If answering email, do it once, at most twice, daily.
- If texts arrive, set aside a time to deal with them, then leave those that follow until the next day. Don't use instant messaging! It keeps you in a state of constant tension, very destructive to your Spleen capability.
- If cleaning or tidying the house, set aside a period of time to do it. After doing it for that period of time, move on to something else.
- If exercising at home, don't stop to tidy a table, or improve a room's layout: just exercise!
- Read one thing at a time.
- If cooking, unless you are a master-chef, aim to do one thing at a time.

Of course, this is easier said than done. I too have had small children around me, demanding attention when I needed to complete work!

When you are harried, worried, trying to out-think circumstances, your Spleen, and your digestion, will work less well. What does that mean?

- Less energy: tiredness
- Tendency to snack, or poor appetite
- More inclination for coffee, caffeine, chocolate

- Tendency to breathlessness or sighing
- Diarrhoea or loose stools
- Desire for sweet or junk food
- Sleep disturbed
- Skin gets drier; less healthy
- Lips crack or dry
- Growing irritability

The above symptoms occur because, in health, your Spleen transforms what you eat and drink into what your body needs, sending it to your Liver, Lungs, Heart and blood vessels.

If your Liver doesn't receive what it needs, your sleep will become less refreshing, you will get headaches or feel 'out-of-sorts' and irritable, your digestion will be disturbed, with distension, burping and loose stools. Furthermore, your skin will lack tone, flexibility and colour.

If your Lungs don't get what they need, you will feel breathless and tire easily.

If your Heart doesn't get what it needs, you won't get far!

Eventually, as the Spleen fails to move fluids around, they get stuck. That could mean oedema, starting in your feet, ankles and legs, and the accumulation of fluids which lead on to phlegm. Your Lungs should send stuff *down*, but if your Spleen works poorly, that rubbish will accumulate, giving your catarrh, phlegm and unwanted gunk in your lungs, throat and nose.

Your Spleen energy has other functions too. In health it should send clear energy upwards and take rubbish downwards. What that means in health is that your thoughts are clear and your voice strong and not disturbed by gunk. Also, by sending energy upwards, it holds things in place, specifically the organs in your abdomen. When Spleen weakens, you get the onset of a large belly, hanging forwards and out. As your internal organs descend, they become less efficient, and you need to rest more, what with the added bulk. So the whole apparatus becomes less efficient, your energy suffers and your spirit weakens.

This often happens insidiously, so that you hardly notice it until you see old photographs of yourself.

Your Spleen energy is susceptible to worry, over-thinking. What does this mean? For example:

- Continually thinking about the same problem or person, even if not worried about it

- Brooding over the past

- A constant state of anxiety

- Obsession or obsessively thinking about something

- Feeling 'bothered' about something all the time

- Continually studying

- Working mentally all the time, rather than using your body to work or to exercise

- Long periods of concentration, especially when tired

The Chinese observation was that the kind of worrying you do will affect your body in different areas:

- If you worry too much, it will affect your chest area

- If you think too much, it is more likely to affect your stomach and abdominal organs.

So too much studying, or too much mental work will tend to 'knot' your intestines (for example, this can lead to irritable bowel disease) whereas just worrying leads to poor breathing habits with the accumulation often of phlegm and, eventually, bad circulation.

Another way of seeing why this happens is that worry tends to make people bend forward or hunch over their chest, blocking easy breathing. Studying means absorbing, which symbolically means we are asking our bodies to swallow and digest information and ideas. Too much study means we have reached our limits and our digestion cramps up to prevent more being forced into it!

However, to distinguish between worry and over-thinking is not always easy.

## Hidden Emotions and Memories

Lastly, sometimes phlegm represents a problem or circumstance in your life.

It may be a certain way of thinking you have – perhaps a rigidity – or an experience or subject which you don't like to think or talk about. This could be blocking your development as a person, stopping you from moving on.

It is almost as if you've wrapped up the emotional issues surrounding the subject and dumped them in your body, which conceals them as phlegm.

Sorting this out is uncomfortable. Talking about it may make you anxious: worried.

You fear the consequences of revealing a side of yourself of which you are ashamed. You worry that doing this may destroy or change a valuable relationship with someone, especially the person to whom you tell it.

If this applies, revealing it could change your life.

Usually this is for the better. Literally, you get the weight off your chest. You become more free.

## Summary

- You may think your thoughts are unimportant in producing phlegm. This chapter is first because it is *so important*.

- Your tendencies to worry, obsess, over-think, all weaken this vital function represented by your Spleen.

- Weakening your Spleen makes you wide open to phlegm.

*The next chapter explains how **what** we eat and **how** we eat it also lead to phlegm.*

# Chapter 4 - Your 'Spleen', Nutrition and the Environment

With good digestion and the right foods, you get less phlegm, often none. Chapter 3 explained how thoughts, emotions and working or living practices can harm your Spleen and lead to greater susceptibility to phlegm formation.

Taking life at a more measured pace can ease your digestion and reduce phlegm, *unless you eat and drink the wrong foods*.

*How* we eat can be as important and as *what* we eat. Nowadays, most people recognise the ill-effects of bad eating habits, such as:

- eating too quickly, stuffing food down
- snacking or 'grazing' continuously
- eating while working
- working while eating
- snatching food 'on the go'
- returning to work too quickly after eating
- swallowing without adequate chewing

- arguing or getting angry while eating
- worrying while eating
- reading while eating
- eating while driving or working machinery
- taking heavy exercise immediately after eating

The same goes for drinking.

Ideally, when we eat we should be calm, unhurried and relaxed, able to take time over it and then take a little light exercise afterwards, such as a short walk. Good company helps us to slow down. Regular childhood meals in a comfortable, familiar and social environment are highly conducive long-term to good eating habits and better digestion.

What about eating alone? Do you read something (paper, magazine, Kindle) as you eat – or watch a video? If so, at least half your mind will be on what you are reading or watching.

The result is that you usually eat faster than you should and take more food than you need, or put more in your mouth and swallow it before properly chewing it.

What happens then? Food takes longer to break down in your stomach and small intestine; you take longer to absorb it into your blood and feel replete. If it takes longer to make you feel replete, you'll keep eating until your stomach is 'stuffed'!

Now, through not chewing on the one hand, and over-eating on the other, you've skewered your Spleen! Doing it occasionally may not matter: doing it often does matter, and the result is that

- you have less energy than you should
- you may feel a little dizzy on rising quickly
- you don't concentrate so well
- your waist tends to expand

- you start getting phlegm!

As we age, our bodies become less reliable and more inefficient. The worse your eating habits and your food and drink are, the faster you age, the more quickly your body succumbs to disease and, among other things, the quicker you get phlegm.

Whereas once, when young, you could eat a huge ice-cream followed by a beer and feel fine, as you age you'll find that you get indigestion quickly followed by mucus then phlegm. That phlegm may appear as more mucus in your throat or nose, or obstructing your vocal chords, so every time you want to speak you have to clear your throat.

Your digestive tract is in contact with the outside, both at either end of it (mouth and anus) and then along its walls, through which nutrients are absorbed into the blood. Until so absorbed, food passing through you is not yet part of you: it remains 'foreign'. How your stomach and intestines react to this foreign matter often reflects how you react to life. (The reverse is certainly true! When constipated, I am less open to the world.)

## Food for Phlegm

Over thousands of years, the Chinese worked out which kinds of food tend to increase phlegm.

*A weak Spleen opens the way for damp and eventually **phlegm** to accumulate.*

So, in addition to teaching yourself to eat in the right way and not the wrong way, consider *what* to eat.

Foods that can weaken the Spleen are:

- foods that are cold or chilled when eaten

- foods with a cold energy (for more on this, see below, and http://www.acupuncture-points.org/cold-foods.html)

- raw foods, ie uncooked, including most fruit and salads or vegetables eaten raw
- cold, chilled or ice-cold drinks, including alcoholic drinks

Foods that have a cold energy are said to have a cooling effect even if eaten warm or cooked. They include many vegetables and fruit, and are even more cooling if eaten uncooked, raw or cold. See the link above for more on this kind of food.

So, as regards what you eat, to reduce the likelihood of phlegm, start eating food *warm*.

This contrasts with foods that have a warming or heating effect, which include meat and spices. Not everyone eats meat, too much of which can be over-heating, (and Heat in the body is also a possible cause of Phlegm, when body fluids are heated and dried).

Again, what are the typical symptoms of a weak Spleen, as noticed over the centuries by Chinese medicine?

- tiredness
- lowered appetite
- preference for lying down
- pale complexion
- weak digestion including runny stools
- distension in your abdomen after eating
- pale tongue

If you have these symptoms, add spices to what you eat. The best spice for this is raw ginger (not ginger powder, which is too heating). You only need a little. Pour boiling water over a few thin slices in a mug, wait until it is cool enough to drink, then sip it from time to time.

[But – before going into particular foods, a reminder! How

and when you eat and how much you eat are all equally important in the production of phlegm.]

- Eat slowly, *chewing well*, in an unhurried, relaxed environment

- Eat regularly, not snacking between main meals

- Sit down and take time to eat, three to five times in a day

- *Do not over-eat!* Over-eating harms your Spleen especially if done regularly or when you are tired e.g. late at night.

- *Under-eating* harms the Spleen. Fasting for too long means the Spleen cannot do its job and your tissues become under-nourished, further straining your Spleen's resources

While cold foods weaken your Spleen, which then becomes less able to remove phlegm, there are other foods which are either hard to digest or which easily lead to phlegm formation:

- Dairy foods often increase phlegm. These are made from cows' milk and cream: yogurt, ice-cream, single and double cream, creme-fraiche, cheese etc. Some people have genes that accommodate dairy food, but many do not. Of course, many dairy foods are eaten *cold*, (eg yogurt, ice-cream, cream, cheese, milk), compounding the problem. In my experience, milk from goats and sheep is easier to digest but may still increase phlegm. Tip: to make milk easier to digest, put a slice of onion in a saucepan with the milk. Heat the saucepan – not so much that the milk boils – until it is pleasantly warm to drink. Drink that. Yes it may taste different, but enzyme action from the onion makes the milk more digestible: *this does not work for everyone, however!* If you are determined to take dairy food even though it increases phlegm production, you should investigate the market for enzymes which, taken beforehand, supply what your body lacks to digest this food. See if they help!

- Sweeteners, including sugar, honey, molasses and artificial sweeteners. As babies nourished by breast milk we have a natural liking for the sweet taste, and in Chinese medicine, the sweet taste is 'good' for the Spleen. But by 'good' they did not mean sweeteners, sugars, honey etc: they meant foods that released their sweetness only after chewing (for example whole grains taste sweeter as mouth enzymes break them down during chewing) or foods that benefited healthy muscular tone, whether or not the food tasted sweet (examples include proteins such as meat – beef, lamb, etc).

- Sweet foods, like bananas, corn, potatoes and foods made from wheat. These quickly turn into sugar when digested: all weaken your Spleen energy.

- Here's a really interesting observation from Chinese medicine, that supports and is supported by modern findings. Perhaps you didn't take it in properly in the foregoing paragraph! Food that turns easily into sugar in your blood-stream leads to many diseases. Mostly these are high-carbohydrate foods ('high carbs') and include junk foods, mentioned again below, and most grain-based foods. In modern thinking, these lead to insulin resistance, harbinger of many, if not most chronic disease, not least obesity. These foods, in Chinese medicine, really damage your Spleen function. You may well say, but what about all the rice they consume?! Indeed, but there have been a few changes in lifestyle over the last 2500 years! Many of us in 'developed' countries have masses of food available and we eat it all the time, especially the foods that appeal to our increasingly sweet teeth.  Such abundance was relatively unknown 2500 years ago, and until recently people people fasted regularly, whether they liked it or not.  Also they lived

hard lives, often short and violent, or outside in all weathers
to farm the foods they needed, sell them, buy them, or run
after or away from people who wanted their foods, land or
resources. Life was different! Foods that turn into sweet-
tasting food damage your Spleen and the result for many is
damp and phlegm. *Indeed, obesity is considered by many to be
a form of phlegm.*

- What about rich food? 'Rich' means greasy or fatty food, also
sugars and dairy foods. Traditional festivals were often when
people rejoiced in the riches of their land, and preparing and
eating rich food was part of the fun. The rest of the year they
probably ate much simpler fare. Many people now have the
resources to enjoy rich food all the time. If they take little
exercise their bodies cannot burn off the calories (mainly
represented by the sweet foods) so they put on weight. If
their weight gain occurred overnight they would recognise
why it happened! Of course, we need fats in food, which the
Chinese don't seem to have forbidden, but of course they ate
the whole food. (And sometimes their appetites became
somewhat jaded, like ours! John Blofeld in his book the
'Wheel of Life' tells the story of how he was invited to a
famous Beijing restaurant in the 1920s where the grill had
apparently never been cleaned in hundreds of years,
hence able to impart complex flavours the customers
craved. We can safely say that the foods cooked there would
have included huge amounts of saturated fats, probably
many carcinogenic in modern view!) At any rate, naturally
occurring fats in themselves do not harm the Spleen.

- Stuff in foods or foodstuffs which only over time do we
realise affect us adversely. Whether from increased use of
herbicides, fungicides, pesticides, antibiotics and artificial
fertilisers used in intensive farming, or from epigenetic
reasons or additives to make food look or taste better or to

last longer, people believe they have become intolerant or 'sensitive' to many foods. Symptoms experienced vary widely but often include symptoms of Spleen deficiency. A food that increases your phlegm might be no problem for me, and vice versa. The older you get and the more carefully you experiment and observe how your body behaves, the more you will discover which foods affect you unfavourably.

- Foods that are 'junk': pre-prepared, often over-flavoured and under-nourishing, containing preservatives etc

- (PLUS ... listed above ... cold, raw, chilled, iced food/drink ... !)

## The Environment and how we enjoy it

Many of us live insulated from nature. Nature can be cold, damp, wet, hot, dry and windy. With central heating and air conditioning, double glazing and damp-proofing, we can observe it but, it would seem, be unaffected by it. But!...

- the bus or train we ride in is a wonderful source of drafts (Wind) as doors open and close;

- sneezing (Wind) in confined spaces spreads illness;

- well-insulated rooms become Damp, with stale air;

- air-conditioning throws cold air (a source of Cold and 'Wind-Cold') at us;

- central heating and electric fires create Dryness;

- global warming is visiting all of us as our atmosphere becomes hotter and less tolerable in many countries, leading to increases in symptoms of Heat.

(For more on Wind, Damp, Cold, Dryness and Heat,

visit http://www.acupuncture-points.org/external-causes-of-disease.html)

Whereas once people suffered from Damp because they worked for long hours in water, fishing or in rice fields, now we have moist rooms in our care-homes and hospitals.

Also, we swim! Formerly, swimming was done mainly in warm climates and by children, or by adults to cool themselves and to fish. Now we swim for a while then loll in the sun in our swimming costumes to dry off in the breeze; sources of Damp and Wind, sometimes also Cold.

The picnic, once an occasional pleasure on rare, hot days (at least, rare in the United Kingdom) is now enjoyed on cold days on cold wet hillsides, when probably our forbears would have taken care to find somewhere protected from the wind, and possibly eaten while standing: they had more awareness of the dangers of damp.

Our Spleen is adversely affected by Damp. We experience dampness when we work in offices or confined spaces even if they are air-conditioned. Old buildings are often damp, especially in basements, even if warm. Some countries or areas are naturally damp, subject to heavy rainfall or regular flooding.

Exercise can make us damp, from perspiration or from air in the gyms where we work out, or from the changing rooms before and afterwards. Many people after exercising in a gym then go home still wearing their damp, sweaty clothes before they shower and change into something dry. Wearing damp clothes when not vigorously generating heat makes the Spleen more susceptible to imbalance.

*For example, I used to cycle to see infirm patients in their homes. Returning one day from such a visit, I got caught in a downpour. It had been a hot day when I started, so I had taken no raincoat. I got drenched. Cycling back after the downpour began to dry me. On arrival at my clinic, I decided I was dry enough and did not need to change, so I immediately started to see patients without changing into dry clothes.*

*The next day I woke feeling crippled by back pain and stiffness. Beginning to move around eased it a bit, and after a warm bath it was much better. It remained better until I had spent 30 minutes sitting talking to a new patient, when the pain and stiffness returned. Movement and heat helped, but every time I spent more than 15 minutes sitting still or lying, the problem returned.*

This was a classic case of Damp invasion, because the stiffness and pain occurred exactly where my skin had remained damp after the downpour.

*(How did I clear it, you may ask? There are many forms of treatment. In fact I took a homoeopathic remedy which cured it in 15 minutes. However, I only realised I needed it when prescribing the same remedy for another patient with a sore and stiff back also caused by cycling the previous day in the same downpour!)*

This was a classic case of being unable, when sick, to observe myself rationally. No doubt this would never happen to you?

At certain times of life we make ourselves more susceptible to the elements. Fashion often dictates that we wear less than we should for health. Clothing is a vital way to prevent invasion by damp. Women make themselves susceptible to Damp invasion by wearing light or revealing clothes during inclement weather: they look wonderful but may weaken their Spleen.

However, some men do this too, by wearing ridiculously little clothing in cold and snow: definitely a macho thing!

The Damp, and often Cold, to which they expose themselves, makes it harder for the Spleen to keep them well.

At certain times of life, people wear less: for example, girls wear thin skirts when playing sports even in cold weather.

Women in general are thought in Chinese medicine to be more susceptible to Cold and Damp during their monthly periods, especially at puberty. At or after childbirth, they should be careful to keep warm and to take time to recover their energy, not least because they have breast-feeding and carrying babies ahead of them, for both of which they need a healthy Spleen energy. But also, having just delivered the baby, the vagina is more susceptible to cold and damp.

In Chinese medicine, many cases of pelvic inflammation and abdominal discomfort start with Damp which invades during puberty or at or soon after childbirth.

Probably giving birth in water is a possible cause too. Water is Damp – obviously! – whatever its temperature, and over many hours during labour, energy is used up: lowered energy makes you more susceptible to invasion by Damp.

One should also realise that high levels of libido tend to make people wear less, and/or expose themselves more. This is often more noticeable in women at certain times in their monthly cycle, but it applies to men too at any time. Wearing less clothing potentially makes them more 'open' to invasion by Damp – and Cold.

What happens when Damp invades from the outside, through the skin?

Chinese medicine has noted the following symptoms connected with Damp invasion:

- Stiffness

- Soreness

- Slowness to get moving: a sense of heaviness

- Lack of appetite

- Abdominal distension, all the more so when pre-menstrual

- Nausea

- Tongue has a sticky, thick coating

- May want more sweet food

- If Damp combines with Cold, continued movement and warmth temporarily benefit the stiffness

*Dampness easily leads to fluid accumulation. Fluid accumulation supplies the perfect opportunity for phlegm to form!*

Typical symptoms of chronic Spleen deficiency are a poor appetite, loose bowel movements, inability to eat large meals, shortness of breath, fatigue, poor concentration even on everyday activities, and a quiet voice. Their tongue is pale and shiny, with a slightly sticky coating. Their pulse, to an acupuncturist, would feel weak and soft, particularly in the Spleen position on the wrist.

## Summary

Phlegm is 'made' by your Spleen when it is weakened. You weaken your Spleen by

- emotions, worry, hurry, frustration, anger …
- taking food at irregular times
- eating without awareness
- not chewing properly: eating raw or cold foods/drinks
- eating foods and drinking liquids with 'cold' energy
- over-eating or under-eating
- eating the wrong foods (dairy food, sweet food, food that is too rich, food that was 'treated' during manufacture)
- allowing yourself to be invaded by Damp and Cold

*The next chapter is on the subject of your **Lungs**. Whereas the experience of Chinese medicine is that your Spleen, when weakened, is unable to prevent phlegm production, (so we shorten this by saying that your Spleen 'makes' phlegm,) the spaces 'ruled' by your Lungs are where the phlegm ends up. Hence your Lungs 'store' your phlegm.*

# Chapter 5 – Your Lungs and your Respiration

Poor breathing gives you phlegm.

In Chinese medicine, (perhaps not surprisingly) breathing comes under your **Lung** energy.

If your lungs are working well, their rhythmic movement keeps your airways clear and, if phlegm accumulates, they move it downwards to your stomach and digestion, eventually to be broken up and disposed of through urination. Alternatively, coughing brings it up to be expectorated.

(... so ... expect that, if you are having treatment, eg herbs, to clear phlegm, you will urinate more ... )

Of course, your Lungs have other important functions!

- They exchange oxygen and carbon dioxide, bringing life to your blood to circulate round your body. They 'govern' your respiration and energy.

- This oxygen – in Chinese medicine it is called 'clean qi' – extracted from the air, combines with the heavier nutrients in the blood, extracted from food you eat. Together they create in your chest a bigger kind of Qi – energy – to nourish your body. From the point of view of phlegm, this process is important as when either your Spleen or your Lungs are deficient, phlegm gathers in your chest. Like rubbish dumped on a road, it then itself goes on to prevents efficient movement, slowing everything down still more, leading to yet more phlegm creation, and loss of energy.

- In health your Lungs spread Qi – energy – around the body, *out* to your skin, and push or send it *downwards*. This 'sending downwards' or 'descending' function is important. With tension, excitement, frustration, anger, tight schedules and targets to meet, your energy tends to rise, which you feel as tension in tight shoulders, headaches, grinding teeth, insomnia, and restlessness; also in the desire to snack, to swallow, to bite your lips. These are more or less unconscious ways to stimulate the descending of energy by stimulating your Stomach, which also should *descend* energy – otherwise you feel nauseous!

- You also use the descending power of your lungs when you breathe deeply and exhale, when you meditate or sing or sigh. In each case it can have a calming effect – though I concede that not all singing is calming! If you are tense or cross, take ten deep long breaths to calm yourself down. Or perhaps you smoke, stimulating your Lungs another way? – a tried and tested method for calming feelings of stress!

- This descending function, sending energy downwards, is complemented by the energy of the Kidneys which (in Chinese medicine) accept, then grasp and contain the Qi. From there the Kidneys send clean moisture up to your lungs. As we'll read in chapter 6, if your Kidneys fail, energy and phlegm accumulates above – in your lungs (which can lead to some forms of asthma, for example, when people cannot breathe out properly). Unable to breathe properly, to keep fluids in motion, you get phlegm in your lungs.

- When energy gets trapped in your lungs because they fail to send it down, the natural flow of fluids can be hindered, including the flow of Blood.  An example of what then happens is that blood circulation to your hands worsens (ie you get cold hands) but, from this phlegm point of view, you cough, your chest and lungs feel blocked, and you can become breathless. Phlegm easily collects when there is a lack of breath or rhythmic movement to clear it out – just like dust under your bed, which you don't vacuum often enough.

- As mentioned, your Lungs also push energy outwards towards the skin. In fact, they are said to control the area just under the skin surface, the area that keeps it nourished, moist and flexible. In good condition, your lungs and your skin easily repel disease.  In Chinese medicine your lungs are your first line of defence and play a huge part in maintaining your immunity from disease. If a disease does manage to invade either your lungs or this space between skin and muscles, it blocks the smooth flow of energy and nutrition. This then blocks the circulation of your immune force which slows down or blocks your Lungs (like traffic backing up after an accident). Then you start feeling ill; you start sneezing, feel chilled, perhaps get a headache, become more introspective and so on. When your lungs succumb to disease, phlegm easily collects.

- What about your nose?! Your Lungs 'open' into and out through your nose. With healthy Lungs your nose is clear, your sense of smell is good, and there is just enough mucus to keep it moist and to absorb dust and particles that might otherwise enter your lungs. Conversely, if your Lungs are unable to maintain nasal health, your nose blocks (if one side often blocks it may be a deficiency in the lung on that side), you may lose your sense of smell and, depending on circumstances and the nature of the invading disease, your nose will become more runny or dry or blocked because your lungs cannot regulate the amount of mucus, or 'descend' it properly. If your Lungs are invaded by what is called in Chinese medicine 'Heat' (see chapter 13) the mucus that collects will becomes more concentrated and discoloured, green or yellow: phlegm!

- Typical symptoms of chronic Lung Qi deficiency include a pale, bright and white complexion, frequent colds, clear watery discharges from the nose ('rhinitis'), frequent chills and dislike of the wind especially of *cold* wind, occasional sneezing even when you don't have a cold (this may be caused by air pollutants, allergens etc), slight wheezing or breathlessness, a weak voice, and a mild productive cough with thin white sputum

- For much more on Lung functions, see http://www.acupuncture-points.org/lung-qi.html.

## Emotions and your Lungs

Just as over-thinking and worry affect your Spleen, predisposing it to weakness and therefore making it more susceptible to the formation of phlegm (as explained in chapter 3), your Lungs are affected by disappointment, grief, sadness and worry.

These emotions affect your Lungs in different ways.

- The Chinese noticed that worry, over-thinking, even obsession,  tended to '*knot*' the energy, the symptoms of which appeared as tightness in the chest and tension in the shoulders. This tightness ("Qi Stagnation") made you less likely to breathe freely and deeply, often less willing to show or admit to feelings, more defensive perhaps. The consequence is restricted breathing, sometimes breathlessness or shortness of breath and a tendency to sigh, yawn, or take occasional deep breaths. This, as previously explained, stops the rhythmic movement of energy round your body and the clearing away of rubbish – so things collect, often in the form of phlegm.

- Disappointment, grief and sadness, on the other hand, tend to *deplete or weaken* your Lung energy. The symptoms of depleted Lung energy ('Lung Qi deficiency') include a weak voice, or possibly speaking loudly at the start of sentences, tailing off to a quieter or feebler voice at the end of the sentence; tiredness and fatigue; a preference not to speak unless you have to; occasional cough – which may, if the emotional impact continues for a while lead to the need to clear your throat every time before you speak; shortness of breath, meaning that on exertion you often have to stop to catch your breath; a much whiter and shinier facial complexion than normal; occasional unexplained spontaneous perspiration during the day; aversion to cold conditions (cold water, cold food or drinks, cold wind, weather or  rooms, exacerbated if not wearing enough), and increased susceptibility to coughs and colds (because as your Lung energy weakens, it cannot spread your defensive energy round sufficiently); tongue is paler than usual. With insufficient Lung Qi, there is insufficient energy in your chest, which can lead to poor circulation in the hands (cold hands), poor self-image and posture. This can lead on to Qi stagnation in the chest, leading to tension and tightness as explained above; and the easy accumulation of phlegm.

## How to relieve the problems of deficient Lungs?

1. Realise that disappointment, grief and sadness take time to recover from and ...
2. ... meantime you have to continue life somehow.
3. As these emotions sap your energy, do something daily to move it. One of the best ways is through exercise. Try

walking, running, skipping, climbing hills, cycling, a sport of some kind ... anything that makes you breathe deeply and lose your breath for a while. That forces energy and oxygen round your body which raises your energy levels. This compensates for that lost through your emotions. (You will benefit even more if your lungs learn how to be more efficient – see below.)

4.  Light. Daylight, from the sun (!) is best, whether winter or summer. Extreme latitudes in winter receive little sunlight, but the air is often cleaner out of doors so learn to enjoy it. If where you live gets very little sunlight for months on end, whatever latitude you inhabit, buy a lamp giving you daylight – light with the same wavelength as day/sunlight. Sit in this light for as long as possible daily. Note – this does not mean you need a suntan, so beware harsh rays of sun tan lamps which can burn you. Pay attention to the instructions! Though not as good as clean air, light is very yang so has many benefits. For example, sufficient sunlight increases vitamin D which boosts immunity and helps to strengthen your bones.

5.  Your Lungs also 'rule' your skin. Sunlight in moderation boosts skin – and your – health.

6.  Company may not be what you want – or perhaps you want only certain company. Still, spending time with other people convivially is another way to move Qi around. Although you may feel desolated and sad again when you return home afterwards, the right company keeps you in touch with the world, when you may otherwise be inclined to turn your face away from it. Also, in company you may lose yourself, whereas in counselling or therapy, which some may recommend, the emphasis is on you personally.

7.  Arrange to have some form of physical hands-on therapy. It could be body massage, shiatsu, head massage or reflexology, for example. These 'skin' therapies give you

direct physical contact, another way of moving Qi round your body or between you and someone else.

8.  Food. If your Lung energy is low because of emotional costs, compensate with warming food, especially spicy food. Spicy food benefits the Lungs, though not if taken in excess: for example, if you take so much that it makes you perspire, you are probably taking too much.

9.  Sleep. Sleep more. A symptom of Lung Qi deficiency is tiredness. Sleep is restorative.

10.  Rest. Don't push yourself too hard. Give yourself permission to rest more.

11.  There are therapies with specific means to ease and stimulate Lung Qi, acupuncture for example. A few sessions may help to raise your spirits and help you to see your way forward.

## Posture

Any posture that restricts easy breathing will tend either to deplete Lung energy or, eventually, to cause Lung Qi stagnation.

- When worried, anxious or sad, you naturally stoop.

- Working at a desk often inclines you not to sit upright.

- Working in confined spaces makes you stoop.

- Cycling with drop handle bars crunches up your lungs.

- When driving vehicles you slump; bad for your back but also for your chest.

- Watching television from low chairs puts you in a poor posture, and means you don't move for long periods. With no need to breathe deeply your lungs function less efficiently. Often you eat in the same position which confines your stomach and intestines: as your stomach fills it presses up against your diaphragm, further reducing lung space.

- Lying in bed to read, watch television or play computer games also scrunches you up. Consequently you don't move much, preventing your lungs from their easy rhythmic movements that could keep you in good health.

*What can you do to reduce bad posture?*

- If sitting, do so with your bum at a higher level than your knees, and your feet side by side flat on the floor or with the heels slightly raised
- If sitting for long periods, time yourself and get up to walk around a bit every 20 minutes.
- Cycle with upright handlebars! Or make sure you get off your bicycle to walk from time to time.
- Get back-posture support when driving and don't drive for too long without stopping. A good rule is to take a walk every half-hour, or swap with another driver, if you can.
- Reduce the hours you watch TV! Go and play a sport that makes you run and jump and breathe deeply, or take up singing in a choir, or join a debating society or go walking …
- Or learn yoga or Tai Chi or Pilates

Believe me, your health will improve and you will get less phlegm! The Chinese saying that phlegm is formed by the Spleen but stored in the Lungs will have less purchase if your lungs are in excellent condition.

Your Lungs are weakened by Cold and Dryness. So if you like snowy conditions, i.e. cold and dry, and have Lung deficiency, keep warm when not active outside.

Your Lungs are weakened by Dryness on its own, too. Air

conditioning, central heating and car space heating all easily dry the air. Take care to have something to provide humidity. If you don't, your body may respond by increasing mucus production, itself potentially a source of phlegm. Alternatively, the dryness will weaken your Lungs making them more susceptible to invasion by infection – another source of phlegm!

## Air quality

Particles in the air should be filtered out in your nose and throat, ending up as mucus swallowed and eventually excreted. Unfortunately, particles easily find their way to your lungs where, collected in mucus, they accumulate to form phlegm.

- Particles from diesel smoke are now recognised as a cause of various respiratory diseases.

- Wood and coal fires produce huge amounts of air particles. Out of doors these are quickly blown away. Indoors, they may end up in your lungs.

- Smoking anything, whether cigarettes or e-vapes or social drugs, sends particles to your lungs.

- Dirty working environments where air is not filtered properly or circulates too slowly lead to dangerous levels of air toxins.

- Concerns about energy loss have prompted architects to design air-tight buildings. These may keep the heat in, but they also keep in old, much-breathed air the oxygen content of which gradually reduces as it is breathed. In effect, you breathe dirty, used, air.

- Cooking in enclosed spaces releases many carbon and other particles into your kitchen and then into your lungs.

- Building, manufacturing and farming can release dangerous chemicals and dirt into the air.

If possible live and work in a good supply of fresh, clean air! At night open the window (unless your open window exposes you to traffic fumes or thieves etc.)
  *Unclean air increases the likelihood of phlegm in your body.*

## Air Quantity and Lung Efficiency

You might think that more air would be better, especially if good quality.
  Maybe not!
  Just as too much food overloads your system, too much air may *decrease* your lung efficiency !
  When, after taking the advice in this book, your phlegm improves, learn breathing techniques to make your lungs work more efficiently. These improve your lung function and help your body learn better ways to metabolise oxygen, which improves your general health, your immune system and your ability to cope with stress and PHLEGM!
  Learn more about them with yoga (pranayama) or from reading books such as 'The Oxygen Advantage' by Patrick McKeown. After you've read and practised what he preaches, widen your lung experience by practising what Belisa Vranich teaches in "Breathe: The Simple, Revolutionary 14-Day Program to Improve Your Mental and Physical Health".

## Summary

- Your Lungs in Chinese medicine are said to circulate energy everywhere in your body: in your arteries and veins, through your organs, brain, skin and muscles and along your acupuncture channels. Everywhere!

- When this energy ( – a better name for it is Qi, pronounced *TCHEE! – )* moves, it carries blood to repair your body and then carries away waste products. Maintaining good levels of Qi throughout your body helps to move fluids and stop phlegm from gathering.

- Exercise and company make you move and breathe better.

- Light is a form of yang energy that raise the spirits, especially sunlight. Get out into it, let it play on your skin (also ruled by your Lungs) and feel the benefit.

- Posture!

- Air pollution! Smoke! Fumes!

- Sleep and rest!

- *Breathing properly gives your more vitality, a clearer brain, healthier skin, more lustre, better immunity. Oh... and a more joyous attitude to life!*

*The next chapter covers your Kidney energy, vital for centering your life, acting as an anchor for your emotions, filtering out phlegm and helping you renew yourself.*

# Chapter 6 - Your Kidneys: the other part of fluid metabolism

The concept of your **Kidneys** in Chinese medicine goes far beyond the concept of the kidney organs in Western medicine. They are responsible, in Chinese medicine, for guarding your life essence, which comes from your parents and which lays out your vitality throughout life.

This chapter explains where, in Chinese medicine, you get your yin and yang from, so bear with me for a little more theory.

This essence looks after your maturing process and your resilience. It is used up as you age. When your body has to sustain injuries or illnesses beyond its immediate capacity, it draws on this deep source, doled out by your Kidneys.

Essence also governs fertility, virility, and to a large extent what is called your 'marrow', the 'fat' that maintains your spine, brain and bones. In good quality it leads to a healthy brain organ, governing thinking, concentration, memory, originality, hearing and sight. If this precious substance is depleted, your brain-power diminishes and your bones become more brittle, conditions now associated with ageing.

From this essence your Kidneys fashion your Yin and Yang energies. This means they are responsible, along with your

Lungs, for fluid metabolism (the actual words describing this are 'transforming and transporting of Body fluids').

Although this process occurs throughout the body, it is mainly in the lower abdomen that we see it in action. Here, the kidneys filter and sort fluids into waste (urine) and re-usable. The power to do this derives from Kidney Yin but the process is more due to Kidney Yang. Splitting it up this way may seem unnecessary, but it helps to clarify what happens and makes it easier to diagnose problems if they occur. For more on this see http://www.acupuncture-points.org/kidney-function.html.

In the lower abdomen you have your small intestine, your large intestine, your kidneys and your bladder. Together these maintain a healthy fluid balance in your body. Your intestines extract fluids from food passing through, and the kidneys maintain balance, storing urine – waste – in the bladder.

Additionally, as explained in chapter 5, your Lungs 'descend' fluids. Some of these 'Lung' fluids are sent to the bladder for excretion and some, after purifying, are sent upwards again to moisturise your Lungs.

As explained in Chapters 3 and 4, your Spleen also transforms and transports, but this is of food essence and Blood. The specific function is Spleen *Yang*. Guess where this Yang comes from? Your Kidney Yang energy!

That Kidney Yang energy supplies Heat too, used by all your organs to do their business and to keep you warm. If this Yang Heat is weakened, your metabolism slows, your organs work less efficiently, and you have lower physical and mental vitality: you get cold, tired and/or depressed.

One other side-effect from lowered Kidney Yang is the gradual build-up of fluids. These can appear in symptoms of Damp, or as oedema. This build-up of fluids makes you more susceptible to phlegm.

Phlegm from Kidney deficiency sometimes peaks at dawn.

Yang energy can be damaged by strong Yin factors, such as

Cold or large quantities of fluid. This form of Cold occurs when you let yourself get cold to the core, perhaps when you wear too little and/or are exposed to cold conditions and then cannot recover quickly.

For example, if you are exercising vigorously in the cold, and stop to rest without covering up, you will chill down. If you can warm up again quickly, either from more exercise or from a warm bath, there may be no harm, but if not, your Yang energy may become depleted. This leaves you open to invasion by other pathogenic factors, and with weakened digestion (Kidney Yang supports Spleen Yang), recovering is further delayed. In due course, you will develop signs of cold in your Kidneys, including low back pain, loose stools, sore periods and pain in your abdomen or symptoms of cystitis (remember the old lady mentioned in chapter 2?), which feel better for warmth.

With Cold, fluid metabolism is retarded, so fluids flow more slowly and tend to stagnate, or 'gel': an obvious sign or precursor to phlegm.

Typical symptoms of chronic Kidney Qi deficiency include chronic breathlessness even on slight exertion; frequent panting or wheezing; low back soreness and weak knees; dizziness; tinnitus; pale complexion; coldness both internally and of arms and legs, hands and feet; fear of cold; easy, even spontaneous perspiration; frequent urination including through the night. Tongue is pale, may have teethmarks on the sides, and its coating is shiny. Pulse is deep, thin and weak, especially in the Kidney pulse position on the wrist.

If Kidney Yin deficiency is also present, you get nights sweats (even when the room is cool), flushing (hot flashes, power flashes), thirst, dry mouth, slight pinkness over your malar bones on your face; your ears, palms and soles may feel unexpectedly hot even if the arms and legs feel cold; anxiety, irritability, restlessness, insomnia.

For more on Kidney syndromes like Kidney Yang, and Kidney

Yin deficiency, see http://www.acupuncture-points.org/kidney-syndromes.html

Summary
Your Kidneys govern:

- your resilience
- your ability to renew yourself
- your ability to warm yourself, to combat Cold
- your ability to balance fluids in your body
- your ability to warm and energise your Spleen yang function that resolves phlegm

*The next chapter describes another way your emotional health has a huge effect on how you cope with phlegm.*

# Chapter 7 - Blocks that stop health

For some of us, this chapter is more important than at first it may seem.

The things we aspire to, and the problems we face getting them, cause frustration. That frustration has been well observed in Chinese medicine and is described as being a form of 'stagnation'.

### Example

*Imagine you are driving happily along on a day out in your big new car; all the traffic lights are green and you waft out into the countryside for a relaxing day by the sea, on your way to meet a friend. You feel comfortable, perhaps excited, about the meeting.*

*You drive down into a dip between the hills when – calamity! – a puncture and a wheel tyre blows out. You steer the car to the side of the road and stop.*

*Nuisance! you ring for help. Bigger nuisance – there's no signal, no chance of making a call!*

*No matter, it's all in a day, you will just change the wheel yourself.*

*You go to get the equipment and the spare wheel. Except there is no spare wheel, and no equipment: this is one of those new cars where no spare wheel is provided, just a compound you squirt through the valve which coats the inside of the tyre and reflates it. Except you had a blow-out, you can put your hand through the hole in the wall of the tyre, and the compound won't work.*

*Now what?*

*Do I detect mild irritation? No longer is the day so jolly! And where you stopped is in the shadow, away from the sun; cold. And time is rolling on with no way to ring your friend.*

*Never mind, flag down a passing car for help.*

*But you came this way to avoid traffic and you were very successful – there isn't any!*

*You'll have to walk uphill until you get a signal. It's a couple of miles either way.*

*Now your mind is beginning to churn: why are car manufacturers so economical – especially in expensive cars like yours? Why aren't cell-phone signals available? Why does your new friend live in such a ridiculously isolated place? Why didn't you bring something to eat? Or a hot drink in a vacuum flask, to warm you up? Or, hang it, some whisky?*

*Your shoulders are tense, your brow is frowning, you are biting your lips – and you've stopped breathing in the comfortable, relaxed, easy way that you were just five minutes ago.*

Let's just take the change in your breathing. If you decide not to walk up the hill to get the phone signal, your breathing will remain shallow. That means your lungs won't be able to relax you, and any phlegm you had in them may produce a cough or wheeze, or make you clear your throat before speaking.

And the irritation you feel will probably prevent the smooth digestion of your breakfast, potentially producing more phlegm to lie in your lungs.

And this was just after five minutes!

*Daily tensions*

Imagine if every day was full of similar impossible frustrations: your breathing would be permanently restricted and your digestion might deteriorate into something like irritable bowel syndrome, with flatulence, occasional tearing pains and unreliable and sometimes urgent bowel movements.

Actually, the best thing you could do, out there in the cold lee of the hill, would be to walk quickly uphill to find both the sun and the phone signal.

This would get you out of breath, push blood round your body, and work off some of the frustration. The worst thing you could do would be to sit and grind your teeth!

In Chinese medicine, you suffered from what is called 'Qi Stagnation" (pronounced *'TCHEE!'* stagnation). Qi, badly translated as energy, stops flowing smoothly, leading to obstructions, the cause being emotional.

*People, colleagues, employees, staff, co-workers*

Another example is when at work you find one colleague or employee who always manages to irritate you or wind you up. Even the sight of him or her may make you tense. Over time, this leads to a state of constant strain for you, certainly enough to cause Qi stagnation!

*Where blocks occur – your channels of acupuncture*

Those obstructions occur along pathways called *channels* or *meridians* in Chinese medicine. (See http://www.acupuncture-points.org/acupuncture-meridians.html)

These channels, it is currently thought, connect different points in your fascia, the smooth sheets of connective tissue that envelop just about everything in your body. They protect and support your internal structures and let muscles and organs ease past one another without friction as you bend, stretch, walk and flex. Meridian theory is sophisticated and enables well-trained acupuncturists to diagnose and deal with a myriad kinds of problem.

What that means is that problems or blocks in one part of the body have potential effects in many other parts of your body. And emotional tensions transmit easily along these channels/fasciae, disrupting the health and processes of the interconnected organs.

*Friction heats, and hot air rises*

Usually Qi stagnation leads to friction which, in terms of Chinese medicine, often increases yang. Yang energy tries to *ascend* (which is why all the six main yang channels *descend* your body, carrying energy down again.)

So Qi stagnation problems rise to the top, leading to tension in your shoulders or head, headaches, fingers that fiddle with things, and phlegm and sinus problems in your lungs, throat and head.

Qi Stagnation is one of the biggest causes of disease in Western society, and increasingly in developing countries where physical labour and bodily movement become less important or possible for work. The rising use of machines, soon to be robots, to do physical work, cleaning, carrying and fetching for us, makes it likely that Qi stagnation will increase as a cause of disease.

It is such a big problem that, for a long time, the page I wrote about Qi Stagnation on my website was by far the most visited. Eventually I wrote a book about it, apparently greatly appreciated by readers: see http://www.acupuncture-points.org/qi-stagnation.html .

So, although this is not a long chapter, it is important because a frequent result of Qi stagnation is Spleen and/or Lung deficiency: your Spleen cannot then do its job, and your Lungs cease to move and disperse energy properly.

As both Spleen and Lungs are involved in the manufacture and storage of phlegm, and phlegm tends to migrate to where there is a concentration of energy, you'll get more of it.

So! What to do?

Long-term, you must sort out the major problems that cause you stress. Of course, stress is impossible to clear from life, and we need to develop a level of resilience to cope with it because the alternative is that, in the long-term, chronic stress leads to chronic disease.

In the short-term, we must develop strategies to dissipate stagnant Qi. Many ways to do this are explained in my book 'Qi Stagnation – Signs of Stress' (http://amzn.to/2lzmw4F). For most people, an excellent thing they can do is to take vigorous exercise – even a fast walk is beneficial! This forces your Qi to move around, so you feel better!

Qi Stagnation can also lead to Qi-phlegm, a so-called 'invisible' or 'non-substantial' form of phlegm, mentioned in chapter 15.

## Summary

- Emotional health leads to physical health
- Strong emotions send energy to places where it gets stuck
- Phlegm goes to where your energy gets stuck: lungs, throat, post-nasal, nose, ears, mouth, head and dizziness

*The next chapter is a brief summary of where you have got to, before going on to describe ways to clear or resolve your phlegm.*

# Chapter 8 - Summarising Phlegm production so far

Phlegm comes from what we put inside us. Phlegm appears because our metabolism enables it to appear – we become susceptible to it.

That may happen because some part of our system is inadequate and/or because it is overwhelmed either by the foods we eat or by other extraneous – external – factors, such as Heat from an infection or the environment, or Cold, perhaps from exposure or from eating too many foods that cool us.

Food we eat is turned into Blood. Fluids and Energy for us to live. That works well if we have healthy Kidney Yang to 'fire up' our digestion and keep all our organs warm, especially

- our Spleen Yang and
- our Lung Yang.

Spleen Yang transforms what we eat into Blood and Energy and transports the Blood round your body, mending and replacing tissues. If it fails, stuff collects.

Your Lungs keep your fluid pathways clear by rhythmically 'descending' Qi. In return your Kidneys send pure water up to moisturise your lungs. Also, because your Lungs control Qi and its movement, they keep the right quantity of fluids circulating smoothly and steadily round your body.

Unless you are overwhelmed by emotions that stop Qi flowing, the Qi continues steadily round your system, circulating your Blood and moving on any rubbish. When Qi gets blocked, eventually (Blood and) fluids don't move.

If fluids hang around, they

- block other fluids and the proper movement of Qi and

- congeal – thicken or

- dry, tending towards a sticky (or sometimes almost powder-like) substance which is hard to shift

(One extra way in which fluids are cleared out naturally is through perspiration and exhalation, mainly controlled by your Lungs. You will recall that your Lungs manage the space between your skin and your muscles. From this, when heated by exertion or fever, heat is normally released in the form or vapour through sweat pores.)

In your lower abdomen, fluids are filtered and sorted by your Kidney and Bladder, ready for excretion.

What could possibly go wrong?!
The short answer is 'Heat' (and sometimes 'Cold'). Where does this Heat come from?

- Stress, usually caused by emotional tension or excitement

- Wrong food or Wrong eating habits

- Infection – classified into Heat, Cold, Dryness, Dampness, Wind or a combination of them

- Yin deficiency

## Stress

A well-known saying in Chinese medicine is that instead of trying to get rid of phlegm with herbs that dissolve it, one should just make sure Qi is moving smoothly. When Qi moves smoothly, phlegm moves on. Hence the importance of not doing anything to halt or slow the natural movement of Qi (chapter 7).

In the West, we recognise stress as a problem, but we don't readily associate physical complaints with it. Chinese medicine did: and has done for 2,500 years.

Stress and emotions that lead to it or are caused by it are recognised in Chinese medicine as major causes of disease. Why? Because they tend to make Qi stagnate.

My book 'Qi Stagnation – Signs of Stress' goes into this in great detail, showing how signs of stress are explained by Chinese medicine and what you can do to help yourself. When you understand stress from an energetic point of view you can see why what you do makes it better or worse.

When Qi is trapped, it easily turns to Heat. Heat warms and concentrates fluids in the body, leading to phlegm.

Stress is a condition we share with animals, and we all deal with it in our own ways. One of those ways is by impeding the flow of Qi through our Lungs and Spleen. When this happens, you create the ideal conditions for phlegm to collect.

Learning to move around sufficiently to promote good breathing habits, and the posture and exercising that helps them, decreases the likelihood of phlegm very considerably, as a side-effect of improving your health generally.

## Food and Eating Habits

I've explained this in chapter 4. Poor food choices and poor eating habits predispose us to phlegm formation. They make phlegm easier to form and harder to shift.

## Infection

Phlegm often accompanies infection. Heat and Damp from the invading infection produce phlegm.

## Deficient Yin

But there is another reason why phlegm can collect: deficient Yin – too little of the cooling, moisturising Yin form of Qi.

Without sufficient yin energy, you get dryness and heat.

This heat is different from that in Hot-phlegm but can contribute to it.

How to understand *deficient yin*?

*Think of it like this. Imagine you are driving across the Sahara desert on a hot day. You get hot, and your car gets hot. What do you do? You turn up the air-conditioning. If the air-conditioning is working effectively, the inside of the car will cool down, but this will use a lot of fuel and the car will remain hot, at least on the outside. The car's engine, working full-tilt, will get very hot, but if its cooling system is working it will continue to function.*

Here the heat is from the outside, a source of *excess yang*.

*Compare that with the same car driving through a cool country on a cold day. Normally, the car's engine would be used to warm air in the passenger compartment without a problem. But if the coolant ran low, the car's engine would overheat, potentially dangerously. Here the heat comes from an internal problem, an internal inability to cool down. This is deficient yin.*

Of course, you can have both! This does happen with some kinds of hot-phlegm, so that already yellow, dry phlegm is further baked by internal deficiency of yin. This makes it harder to cure. It happens mostly in older people who have had chronic phlegm for years and whose bodies are exhausted. Usually, herbs that clear Heat are different from those that supplement Yin and moisturise and cool, in the same way that taking a car out of the sun lets it naturally cool down, but its engine will still overheat unless the coolant is replenished.

This sort of situation is best treated by a professional. Doing it oneself can lead to mis-diagnosis and mistakes. Besides, professionals have knowledge of and access to a far wider range of treatments.

## ROOT AND BRANCH

You want to get rid of your phlegm!
*You must think about it in two ways.*

### Root

The root of the problem is one or more of the following:

- Spleen: the food you eat, your eating habits, your thinking habits and anxiety or *over-thinking*
- Lung: the environment you inhabit, the exercise you take, and how you breathe: also grief and disappointment
- Kidney yang: poor circulation and warmth
- Qi stagnation: the stresses in life
- Yin deficiency: exhaustion of your cooling, moistening ability

### The Branch

This is how phlegm manifests.

Do the right thing and you'll reduce or clear it. But it will return unless you also deal with the root, above.

- Fatigue phlegm
- Damp phlegm
- Cold phlegm
- Hot phlegm
- Dry phlegm

Sometimes root and branch need the same treatment, sometimes different.

Root treatment often needs a fundamental re-think of how you live, plus treatment from a professional – for example for Kidney Yang deficiency – though you can help. These root habits are often hard to change and maintain, but unless attempted, the phlegm will return, or may never go away.

Branch treatment is something that both you and your professional therapist can treat. In fact, often you can do it yourself to a considerable extent. Having read this book, you will try the branch treatments.

Let me just repeat! *You must treat the root cause too!*

*The next chapter explains a wide variety of ways people have used to clear phlegm. Why do some work, and not others?*

# Chapter 9 – General ways to clear phlegm

Normally, dust collected in mucus or by the tiny hairs ('cilia') in your nose is propelled towards your throat. From there it is swallowed, descending to your stomach to be digested and eventually evacuated through bowel action and urination. This protects your lungs from getting clogged up.

However, when you are ill, phlegm does collect in your upper respiratory tract, your nose, throat and lungs.

There are many ways to clear phlegm, some more effective than others.

Advice specific to each kind of phlegm is given in the following chapters, but here is a list of various ways in which your body either naturally or with help clears it, although some methods clear it only for a while.

When you have read later chapters you will realise why some of the methods listed below are *inappropriate* for *your* particular kind of phlegm.

## Do It Yourself

- Cough – usually this is involuntary!

- Hawking it up and expectorating it

- Steam, a vaporizer, or hot moist air (eg hot shower) inhalation to loosen and dilute the phlegm

- Maintaining correct humidity in the environment

- Salty water: various ways to use it to loosen or flush away phlegm in your nose or sinuses. Some involve gargling salty water; with others you sniff up small quantities into a nostril and let the water run back into your throat from where you can spit it out, or by angling your head you get the water to emerge from the other nostril, carrying phlegm with it. Another way to do this is with a 'Neti' pot – but it is very easy to learn to do it without the need for the Neti pot, which is just another way to separate you from your money!

- Warm compresses, eg to the face

- Sleeping with the head well elevated

- Avoiding irritants and pollutants, wearing masks etc. (Irritants include perfume, moulds, yeasts, chemical odours, dust, pet hair or dander and smoke.)

- Changes of temperature, such as when exiting from warm air into cold air, or vice versa

- Blow your nose – gently

- Drinking plenty of liquids which helps to dilute the phlegm, making it easier for your body to deal with. However, this may *increase* your phlegm if you have Tiredness phlegm, Damp or Cold phlegm.

- Voluntary hyperventilation: not recommended unless you know what you are doing

- Yogic breathing practices: need practice

- Avoiding bad food – food that increases or causes phlegm. Surprisingly effective, and only needs a little self-discipline. If you eat the wrong food, (eg too much; junk food; sweet food; cold food; for more see chapter 4! – but also bad eating habits) you can notice more phlegm within a few minutes

- Fresh, cool, clean air is best for Hot phlegm and good for all forms of phlegm unless the air is too cold for comfort (Fatigue phlegm, Damp phlegm and Cold phlegm) or too hot (Hot phlegm, Dry phlegm).

## Needing help

- Massage eg on the back, as in chest physiotherapy: teach a friend to help you, having learned from a physiotherapist

- Postural drainage: as above, get someone to show you how to to this. However, this is a technique used for serious long-term problems such as with cystic fibrosis so may be rather more 'heroic' than you are prepared to face.

## Medication

### Antibiotics

**"Antibiotics are wonderful!"**
But eventually they make your problem worse as your body becomes reliant on the medication, which becomes less effective over time. Increasingly doctors realise the dangers of over-prescribing antibiotics: the bugs mutate and learn how to survive, then when you are really ill, no antibiotic can help.

Then you're back to your own devices, which is where this book may help.

Technically, in terms of Chinese medicine, most antibiotics have a cooling effect, which is why they are effective against infected, highly-coloured, ie 'hot' phlegm. But their secondary effect is to weaken your Spleen energy – probably already weak because otherwise you might not have the phlegm in the first place – which causes more phlegm to collect.

In addition, the antibiotic also destroys the good bugs in your digestion, making you more susceptible to disease. Being cooling in effect, they weaken the natural Yang energy you need to digest food, so you get loose bowel movements, and don't absorb the liquids you need.

So, although I say "antibiotics are wonderful" above, *I don't mean it.*

Chinese medicine contains many amazing formulae which have a similar effect to antibiotics but without the harmful side effects. Not only do they clear the phlegm but they strengthen the Spleen. However, this is where you need either a trained acupuncturist or a Chinese herbalist, who can diagnose your particular condition and treat you accordingly.

The Chinese herbal formulae have antibiotic qualities but also support your digestion.

If you must use antibiotics – which I do NOT advise – then make sure that foods you subsequently eat will repopulate your gastrointestinal tract with beneficial bacteria.

The best foods are green vegetables, very lightly cooked, but everyone will tell you that natural yogurt is best. Well, it isn't! Yogurt and kefir have a very cold quality, detrimental to your Stomach Yang energy, which is why yogurt is often eaten with hot curries: yogurt reduces the heat of the spices. So use yogurt and kefir only if you have Hot phlegm!

Better is warm soup made from miso with a little ginger, or good fermented foods like sauerkraut, natto, kimchi, kombucha and tempeh. Sauerkraut is a name given to cabbage that has been fermented in brine, and kimchi is its Korean cousin.

Kombucha is made using a special yeast culture in tea: easy to make yourself once you have acquired the culture.

Tempeh is a specially fermented form of soya beans. In their fermented form, the beans lose the 'bad' qualities as yet little recognised when eaten raw or liquidised as soya milk.

Even here there is a problem because, for instance, sauerkraut sold in shops has often been pasteurised, reducing its good qualities.

Later, when stronger (i.e.more yang and yin in balance), you can add yogurt and kefir, but just remember yogurt and kefir are both cooling *and* made from dairy foods, which often increase phlegm of the cold, damp sort!

## Expectorants

Expectorants are sold over the counter and contain sugar to give you a little more energy to bring the phlegm up, but also to increase its quantity a little: a curiously perverse way of dealing with it but sometimes very thick phlegm is impossible to expectorate, and making it more bulky and less viscous can help. However, you could just drink warm water infused with ginger which would probably have a similar effect and doesn't load your Spleen with damaging sweeteners.

Many expectorants also contain herbs such as those listed below, but in small quantities, so as to be 'safe'. The herbs may help – but the sugar will not. Better take the herbs, if you know what you're doing.

## Mucolytics

Mucolytics create mucus: hardly what you might think you need! But if they help to thin the mucus they make it easier to expectorate. In effect what they actually do is break down the 'sticky' chemical bonds holding the phlegm together which makes it easier to clear as mucus. They are prescribed by doctors for long-term deep-seated lung problems such as cystic fibrosis and chronic obstructive pulmonary disease (COPD). They must be taken regularly. Taken as prescribed, they are usually safe, but ANY medicine has primary and secondary effects. The latter are usually detrimental: with many mucolytics, the danger is that they break down not just the phlegm but also the walls of your stomach, creating bleeding.

Mucolytics are powerful medicine. Hot water made with a slice of raw ginger has a somewhat similar effect and is much safer. See below for why.

### Antihistamines

Histamines are a form of defence which creates liquids – mucus – and inflammation as your body tries to defend itself against a perceived irritant. The liquids created often occur in your nose or eyes, making them runny. If your health is susceptible, these liquids can become thick, forming phlegm. Here the phlegm is secondary, often caused by infection from some other source happily taking residence in your mucus.

The aim of antihistamines is to stop this at source by obstructing the release of histamines. Some people are very susceptible to histamine reactions, creating misery for them.

Although antihistamines are a boon, they are not a cure. The antihistamine has to be metabolised by your body to excrete it, just like any substance, including medications and herbs.

The problem with medications is that they are often much stronger and less well tolerated than herbs, which are usually less concentrated. The side-effects may be worth it short-term, but long-term they can become insidious and lead you to take other medications to compensate.

I have known patients who, when I saw them, were on up to 15 different medications including a nebulizer. These had gradually been added over a period of years to deal with increasing symptoms caused (in my opinion) originally by the side-effects of anti-histamines.

Caught early, with good acupuncture, for example, many people have overcome their dependency on anti-histamines.

(Note to people interested in homoeopathy: don't get confused! This book explains how to use herbs and foods from a **herbal** point of view. For example, onion, *(allium cepa)* is recommended in this book for cold-type phlegm because its primary effect is warming. If you knew what you were doing, from a homoeopathic point of view, it might be used for hot-type phlegm, or phlegm which is worse in hot environments such as warm rooms. Most people will not have the knowledge or experience to prescribe on this basis – so outside this paragraph, there is virtually no other reference to homoeopathy in this book. To read more about the ideas behind homoeopathy, see http://www.acupuncture-points.org/homeopathy-definition.html)

## Phlegm *suppressants*

These dry your phlegm. I haven't tried them with Dry phlegm, but I have tried them with Cold, Damp and Hot phlegm.

They worked! The phlegm dried up and disappeared, and I could breathe through my nose again!

But there was a serious downside which stopped me from continuing to use them: I got dizzy.

There's an explanation for this in Chinese medicine: briefly, suppressed phlegm doesn't go away, but changes its form.

One of the symptoms of phlegm in its *'non-substantial'* form – ie you can't touch or see it – is dizziness.

I experienced it as dizziness, but you might experience it as mental confusion, or difficulty with co-ordination, eg driving a car. This is more serious than phlegm, and might lead to consequences including falling, or driving accidents.

Anyway, I soon stopped. I do not recommend phlegm suppressants that dry your phlegm and expand your airways. When I stopped taking the phlegm suppressant the dizziness disappeared – but my phlegm returned.

## Herbs, Spices, Foods and other ways of clearing phlegm

### Stimulants

#### Coffee

In terms of Chinese medicine, coffee *(coffea)* seems to stimulate Kidney Yang energy.

So if you feel a bit cold and old, rather depressed and slow, coffee will stimulate your metabolism, making it easier to clear phlegm. For this, it is best taken neat, without sugar, food or milk – not least because sugar and milk tend to increase phlegm; as to food, well, it depends what kind of food! Read chapter 4 on Nutrition.

However, there is a downside: coffee also drains Kidney Yin. Symptoms of deficient Kidney yin take a while to develop, but they include tinnitus, tension, sometimes headaches, jitteriness or a sense of being 'wired' and eventually grey hair; difficulty sleeping, low backache, unusual perspiration – often at night, tiredness, thirst, hearing loss and infertility. Read more at http://www.acupuncture-points.org/kidney-yin-deficiency.html

So do not take strong coffee for phlegm too frequently. If this is the only way you find you can clear it, I suggest *strongly* that you seek treatment from a practitioner of Chinese medicine who will provide acupuncture and herbs to balance your Kidney energies. Incidentally, s/he will also be able to help you to clear your phlegm much faster and more safely than by taking coffee! This will also strengthen your Spleen and Lungs and generally improve your health.

### Pungent foods

#### Cayenne – Chilli

Cayenne *(capsicum annuum)*, also called chilli, comes in various forms and levels of heat. It is a hot, pungent and drying herb, so can be very useful against *cold* conditions and cold phlegm. It generates yang energy and warmth in the body.

As most people know, it makes you sweat so is used herbally to combat invasion by a cold such as 'Wind-Cold' (http://www.acupuncture-points.org/wind-cold.html). It is not, first and foremost, a phlegm-clearing herb, but because it stimulates yang energy in the body, greatly improving the power of your Spleen and Stomach energies, it has a secondary cold and damp-phlegm-clearing effect.

• NOT for use against hot-type or dry-type phlegm.

• supports your body in combating cold or damp phlegm

Part used: the fruit

**How to use**: cayenne comes in various forms; powdered, from your grocer; as an infusion or a tincture (see how to make these in the appendix).

For phlegm, if you just have the powder, put 0.5g in warm water and dissolve. Sip gradually – but use less if the cayenne is very hot, more if not so powerful. If you use too much it will make you sweat, which usually for clearing cold phlegm is counter-productive as sweating cools you down. So use enough to warm you up, but not enough to make you sweat – though it can be a fine line between these two conditions! (On the other hand, if you are taking it for an invasion by Wind-Cold, making you heat up and sweat is exactly what may be needed, demonstrating how herbs can be used in different ways for different purposes.)

Caution: **not for use during pregnancy, nor where there is any inflammation**, for example of the skin, the throat or the bladder. Cayenne is a strong stimulant, so do not overuse.

However, added in small quantities to other herbs when the aim is to clear Cold or Damp phlegm, it provides additional yang-type benefits, particularly where there is tiredness.

---

*Garlic (raw)*

---

Garlic *(allium sativa)* is a food used worldwide. It is very pungent, and in herbalism is also regarded as being slightly sweet and salty. Its main quality is that it is hot and drying. That means that it supports your Yang energy and helps to generate warmth and to clear cold.

That makes it excellent for clearing cold phlegm, but not good for hot phlegm. (Hot phlegm is coloured, ie yellow or green, lumpy or thick, possibly viscous like string; has a strong smell and is usually hard to expectorate. It comes with offensive breath, sore throat, nose or sinuses, and probably with a fever. Your doctor will propose that you take antibiotics though this book offers alternatives.)

If you take it for hot phlegm, it will concentrate and dry it even more, making it harder to clear and tending to increase your sensation of heat. People will argue that garlic's antibacterial qualities will reduce your infection, but this may take time and you may not be really understand how much or whether this is helping your body's natural defences.

Use it for cold phlegm! (This phlegm is colourless, transparent or white, not usually very thick or coloured except possibly on waking after sleep, and often runny, from nose, sinus, throat and lungs. It has no smell, but increases after eating or drinking cold food or too much food, or indeed after any food. See more about this in chapter 12 on Cold phlegm.)

How to take it: remove the papery covering round the garlic clove. Crush the clove and eat it. If eating the clove is too uncomfortable, take it with warm water or, having poured hot water over the crushed clove, let it soak for a while before swallowing the water and the clove. Take up to six cloves a day.

The downside to this is that your breath and skin will smell of garlic! It is these pungent smelly qualities that make it most effective and quick-acting so garlic tablets that have no smell or taste will be less effective as they go straight to the stomach, bypassing your nose, throat and lungs.

Other problems with garlic? It is so strong that it may cause burning in your stomach. In this case, take it with warm water, as explained, or reduce the quantity or size of the garlic clove. In addition, add a thin slice of ginger to the garlic when soaking it. The ginger helps your stomach digest the garlic. Other herbs that may ease your stomach when taken with garlic include cumin and coriander.

What about garlic pearls or capsules? In garlic pearls the garlic is enclosed in a soluble gelatin shell: much more convenient, but as the garlic concentrate was made some time beforehand and reaches your stomach without release of vapour, it is less effective, so you need more of them. Read the instructions on the packet. (Also, you may prefer not to eat gelatin, made from animal sources.)

**Cautions**: garlic is a HOT food!

Too much of it, by overstimulating your Yang energy, may inadvertently drain or reduce your Yin energy. This means that if you have yin deficiency (see http://www.acupuncture-points.org/yin-deficiency.html) or suspect you may be Blood deficient   (see http://www.acupuncture-points.org/blood.html) this herb should be used with great caution, if at all.

Also, because your reproductive health depends so much on your Yin energy, avoid garlic in high dose if you are trying to get pregnant, are pregnant or are breast-feeding, or (being male) suffer from premature ejaculation or spermatorrhea.

If you suffer from spontaneous bleeding, eg nosebleeds or bleeding between menses, both of which are often signs of excess Heat, avoid garlic. As explained, garlic will tend to make hot-type phlegm *worse*, so don't use it for that!

Once your immediate phlegm (cold type!) problem has been solved, you may find that a lower, daily dose of garlic helps keep you fit. It has many other qualities not listed here, highly beneficial for deficient yang conditions, helping immunity and purifying your blood vessels. Long-term use may even incline your metabolism to become less cold, even hot, in which case of course garlic would cease to be useful for phlegm (if you now have hot phlegm!).

Friends must get used to your smell.

*Onion (raw)*

Onion *(allium cepa)* shares many qualities with Garlic, but is not usually quite as strong. Like garlic, onion is hot and drying, so use it for Cold phlegm. It is best taken crushed, raw, or in a little warm water. Taken that way, its pungent qualities help to disperse the phlegm more quickly.

As with garlic, it can produce a burning sensation in the stomach if taken raw. If so, combine it with a slice of ginger root in warm water to make it tolerable.

The same cautions arise as with garlic. However, most onions are not as pungent or warming as garlic so the effect is also less intense on yin or fluid deficiency.

Cooked, onion loses its pungent qualities. Instead, its 'sweet' qualities become more effective, nourishing and strengthening.

If you have phlegm, cooked onion (including shallots, roasted or baked) is a good form of food for most people.

## Horseradish

Horseradish *(rafanus albus)* is a pungent, hot, drying herb: yang in nature. Most British think it is like mustard, to be used with beef, but the herb is much more than that.

Because of its strong warming nature, it is excellent at helping your body clear out cold. This makes it a superb food/herb to stimulate the lungs and digestion (Lungs and Spleen) to dry damp conditions and to warm and expel Damp or Cold phlegm.

It also stimulates the intestines and bladder, meaning that as it gets to work to clear the phlegm you may find yourself urinating vigorously – and your bowels may be stimulated too.

Part used: the root

**How to use**: buy horseradish in the root form, not powder or sauce. The root should be fresh. Use apple cider vinegar to create an infusion, (see appendix for how), leaving it overnight. Or make it into a tincture, or squeeze or crush to extract the juice. Alternatively, grate the fresh root.

If taking the juice, take 15 – 20 drops in warm water, sipped over a few hours.

If taking the grated root, use 2 – 4 g, in warm water.

Tincture: 6 – 12 drops in warm water.

**Cautions**: horseradish is a *hot* herb! Do not use if you have inflammation anywhere, or fever or feel feverish. **Do not use during pregnancy.** Do not use if you are thyroid deficient or hyper-thyroid. Stop if it causes perspiration or diarrhoea.

*Radish (raw)*

Radishes come in different forms: small red radishes are common in the West: in the East, daikon – white radishes are larger and lengthier. With radishes, the skin contains many of the most important qualities.

All radishes are pungent, but unlike garlic and onion, they are slightly *cooling*. Hence they help to clear hot phlegm: yellow, thick, offensive, hard to expectorate, stuck in the nose, sinuses, throat or lungs.

Take sliced, raw, soaked in warm water with a thin slice of ginger. Sip the water, then chew and swallow the radish.

However, they also work well if eaten raw, chewed well. They help to clear the heat and disperse the phlegm.

As with garlic and onion, the Chinese traditionally take fresh radishes regularly as an excellent way to preserve health throughout winter and to ward off disease.

## CHEMICAL

### Colloidal silver

Colloidal silver users claim it can purify water, kill bacteria and sterilise skin. If it has antibacterial qualities it could be used against hot type phlegm. Against cold or damp phlegm it may help very little, if at all.

How to use: read the instructions on the product. Be aware that tests done in 1995 by a herbal distributor on nine different colloidal silver products showed that their quality and concentration varied hugely and that only five of them demonstrated anti-bacterial qualities. Since then claims for colloidal silver have been banned by the FDA and other jurisdictions. In addition, theoretically, overuse can poison you

(but you would need to use a lot for this to happen, and the same could be said for just about anything!)

So, good quality colloidal silver may kill bacteria. This may take the 'heat' out of hot phlegm, possibly leaving you with cold phlegm for which other herbs or foods would be necessary.

## NUTRITIONAL

### Vitamins B6 and Magnesium

I list this combination having seen it being extolled for phlegm management. However, so wide are the individual and combined benefits of these two substances, each essential to human health, that either or both of them could theoretically be proposed for almost any disease.

Together, they help your body manage its metabolic processes. Without them, you would grow sick then die: that is how important they are! If you eat a broad range of foods, freshly prepared, you should get enough of them. That many people need supplementation is a sad reflection on modern nutrition, diet and food habits.

So, as far as phlegm is concerned, make sure you get enough of these two vital substances. If you do not get enough of them, phlegm may be the least of your problems.

### Lemon juice

Lemons are sour and cool, which is why we like cold lemonade in hot weather. This makes them of limited use against cold or damp phlegm. Against hot phlegm lemon juice can help, by cooling and diluting the phlegm. But lemon juice is not a primary anti-phlegm food, though because lemons are also a little astringent (though much less than lemon rind, see below) the juice may help to reduce mucus secretions a little, possibly contributing to a reduction in cold phlegm, in which case take it in warm water!

Because of that astringency, lemon juice can reduce fatigue phlegm, but it does so by tightening up the 'pores', not by increasing your energy. You would need something else for that, perhaps rosemary, for example.

Lemon rind is also sour but much more astringent. Essential oil from the rind has many uses, mainly against hot-type diseases, including hot phlegm.

Dose: *essential oil* – 5 – 10 drops in warm water, sipped, three times a day.

## Vitamin C

Vitamin C (which contains ascorbic acid) is essential for health. It is cooling, so of more use against hot phlegm. However, to be effective, large quantities are needed. As vitamin C is found in fruit, and fruit is mostly cooling, eating plenty of fruit in summer helps to arm your body against hot phlegm production.

But because fruit is cooling, eating too much of it may of itself promote mucus secretion, unless many sour fruits are eaten, sourness having an astringent effect. Increased mucus leads potentially to increased levels of cold phlegm.

So eating too much fruit, or taking too much vitamin C, has a cooling effect and may produce cold or even damp phlegm.

On the other hand, most vegetables, (eg broccoli, cabbage, etc) are less cooling than fruit and contain high levels of vitamin C unless overcooked or not fresh. Increase the number of vegetables you eat, year round: for vitamin C they are your best bet if you tend to be cold.

If you tend to be warm most of the time, eat more fruit, but be aware how damaging the high levels of sugar found in fruit can be if you have any tendency to diabetes.

In general, vegetables are best.

### Chicken broth

Chicken broth is an ancient and prized health food. It is warming and sweet, benefiting the Spleen and Lungs. So this is best for cold or damp phlegm. Against hot phlegm it is much less effective and theoretically could make it worse.

However, in someone exhausted or weakened by a lengthy period of chronic hot phlegm, it may help to renew their energy.

But other treatments would be needed to clear the hot phlegm. Herbal treatment would be fastest.

How to make: there are many recipes for chicken broth/soup on the internet. Buy organic ingredients if you can and cook them very slowly to extract most benefit.

### Honey

Honey is moistening and very sweet, neither particularly hot nor cold. So it particularly benefits dry phlegm. In small, dilute quantities, it provides energy and nourishes the Spleen and Stomach but if you take too much, its sweet nature eventually weakens Spleen and Stomach causing more phlegm.

What that means is that if you are cold, it helps to warm you. If you are hot and exhausted, it re-energises you. But being sweet and moistening, too much will be counter-productive in combating cold or damp-type phlegm.

### Ayurvedic concepts

Although this book mainly explains phlegm from the point of view of Chinese medicine, if you understand Ayurvedic doshas, the following may clarify the differences between the forms of phlegm covered in this book.

|                | Vata | Kapha | Pitta |
|----------------|------|-------|-------|
| Fatigue phlegm | +1   | +1    | 0     |
| Damp phlegm    | 0    | +2    | 0     |
| Cold phlegm    | +1   | +2    | -2    |
| Hot phlegm     | 0    | +2    | +2    |
| Dry phlegm     | +1   | +1    | +1    |

## Tea

No book on health produced in Britain can hope to be taken seriously unless it includes how tea can help.

We're talking here about Indian and Chinese tea including green tea, black tea and all the other forms of tea that have emerged from *camellia sinensis*.

The basic effect of tea is that it is *cooling, bitter and a little sweet* but each kind of tea varies the strength of these three qualities, so the following is very generalised.

- In Chinese medicine, tea is said mainly to affect the Heart, Lungs and Stomach energies. (For 'Stomach', read 'Spleen' as far as this book goes.)

- Its effect on the Heart comes from its bitter quality (and the bitter quality relates to the caffeine and other stimulants it contains). So it tends to raise the spirits.

- Its bitterness also makes it astringent, so on the face of it, it helps to clear or break up phlegm, although its sweetness increases moisture. This moisture can, in susceptible people, lead to more phlegm. This is more likely to happen if tea is taken with milk and sugar.

- Concerning **Fatigue** phlegm, it benefits the Heart and Spirit (as the British have noticed) but being slightly cooling even if drunk warm, and diuretic, it increases urination, which cools you down, making necessary another cup, to the delight of the countries that grow it. Too much tea then overstimulates the kidneys which may have a long-term draining effect on the body.

- When taken black it can help clear **Damp** phlegm in warm climates or in people with good circulation – those with warm bodies! For chilly people with Damp phlegm or in cold climates its benefits are less certain because although it breaks up the phlegm to some extent, it is cooling which is the opposite of their needs, and sweet, which tends to produce moisture, of which they already have a surfeit.

- Since tea is cooling, it is not beneficial for **Cold** phlegm.

- Being cooling and bitter, the effect of which is slight astringency, it helps to clear **Hot** phlegm.

- For people with **Dry** phlegm, being cooling and sweet (ie moisturising) it is usually beneficial unless they are also cold ie have poor circulation. (Even here, you could argue that its effect on the Heart makes it stimulating, but this effect may require many doses, which eventually leads to too much fluid, straining the Kidney energy.)

*The next chapter is the first that explains how to deal with the kinds of phlegm described in chapter 1. Fatigue phlegm!*

# Chapter 10 Fatigue Phlegm and how to deal with it

Have you ever found tears pouring from your eyes, even though you aren't cold, you aren't facing the wind, and you aren't sad or upset?

It seems inexplicable. What makes it worse is that people keep asking what is the matter!

If that's you, this is your chapter! However ...

*... the name of this chapter on 'fatigue phlegm' is not correct!* That is because it covers mucus and other body fluids, not phlegm, or at least, not 'phlegm' as meant in Chinese medicine.

However, the stuff is still liquid, often runny and a nuisance! So this chapter is here because lots of people suffer from it, many doctors don't understand it – and Chinese medicine does.

Also, when you have real phlegm from another cause, eg Damp, Cold, even Heat and Dryness, you may also be tired, with some of the symptoms described in this chapter.

This kind of liquid can certainly come from the nose, but it has cousins! Fatigue phlegm can emerge from almost anywhere:

- mouth – too much saliva; can dribble, embarrassingly, or during sleep

- nose – runny with watery mucus, all the time or frequently or when you enter a new environment, or when cold
- skin – frequent perspiration, even when neither hot nor exerting yourself; just seems spontaneous – without reason!
- urine – you lose it too easily, meaning that you find it hard to control and have sudden emergencies
- eyes – water (lachrimation) occurs too easily, to the point sometimes when others think you are crying
- stools – often watery or mushy, though not diarrhoea

These symptoms occur as your body becomes less efficient and, in terms of Chinese medicine, your Qi is weaker – see below!

If so, you may also have some of the following symptoms:

- slight shortness of breath
- your voice is either already weak or weakens quickly when speaking, and even faster if singing or shouting
- you have little muscular strength, or soon run out of it
- you have low energy reserves – you feel tired, and not much better even after a good sleep
- your appetite may be less than normal; you fill up rapidly; your hunger soon goes when eating
- your stools are 'loose', 'runny': you may find that you get little warning that you need to go
- standing still, or walking slowly, soon tires you

Frequently you have other symptoms too, depending on which 'organs' in Chinese medicine are involved:

- If your Liver is involved then you may find that bright light, from the sun or strong artificial light, is painful in your eyes and it makes them water even more

- If your Heart is involved you get palpitations, pallor, more spontaneous perspiration; possibly some depression

- If your Lungs are involved you probably also have a slight cough, you dislike speaking much, you easily catch colds and you avoid cold conditions if you can – and your nose runs

- If your Spleen is involved, you probably also have a poor appetite, easily get abdominal distension after eating, like lying down, and look pale – and have loose or runny stools

- If your Kidneys are involved, you would have lumbar pain or soreness, your knees in particular would feel weak or unreliable and probably painful, your memory might be poorer, your hearing lessened or with tinnitus, you would urinate frequently but without much force to it and then dribble afterwards or on exertion, and women might have a chronic white discharge from the vagina and probably a dragging sensation in the low abdomen: you would feel cold

If your organs are involved, as explained above, rest and good food might not be enough: you should also seek treatment from someone who understands 'energetic' medicine, such as Chinese medicine, traditional acupuncture.

What is this kind of 'phlegm' and why does it occur?

There is a saying in Chinese medicine that –

### "When Qi is Weak, Fluids leak"

These symptoms are symptoms of Qi deficiency, of tiredness or fatigue.

- You may notice these symptoms when you are tired before

a holiday, when you have been working flat-out to get everything ready before you depart. After a few days' holiday and rest the symptoms improve.

- This kind of fatigue could occur after an illness or shock, or after a period of hard physical work, a succession of disasters or very *draining* experiences including blood loss

- They may appear if you have been under-nourished.

- Some could occur when you lack yang energy in your Lungs or Spleen.

- Or you may notice them in the evening if you have spent the entire day concentrating on work indoors, when you eventually finish for the day, put on your outdoor clothes and go outside, perhaps to go home. There is a fresh wind and perhaps a bright sunset, and your eyes start watering, far more than usual. You may also find you have more saliva, and your nose is more runny than usual.

If you find yourself 'winded' by the breeze, this would confirm that you are suffering from mild Qi deficiency and, literally, fluids are 'leaking'. (As mentioned, technically this is not phlegm as explained in the rest of this book, but slight overproduction of natural mucus.) Were you to walk fast, you might find yourself perspiring, even though you seldom perspire unless exerting yourself heavily.

Your Qi is unable to hold things in place and 'together'. So liquids trickle out.

### How to deal with Qi Deficiency fluids leakage?

Easy!

- Don't work so hard!

- Rest more

- Sleep more. If your work patterns have been such that you are used to just a few hours of sleep, the benefits from increasing the hours you sleep may take time to appear as your body adjusts.

- Speak less – for a while. Talking uses energy. You are supposed to be resting! Take note – teachers, singers, sergeant majors and others who must often speak loudly.

- If you have big time zone shifts on your way to your holiday, take even longer sleeps when you arrive.

- Take things easy!

- Take a holiday!

- Relax more.

- If you are usually bossy and organising in life, let someone else take the initiative for a while.

- Be careful about sudden huge increases in sun exposure. The sun is an immense source of heat and yang energy, so respect it. Don't at first lie out in the sun's rays all day, even with good skin protection. Sleep or rest part of the time in the shade. Increase your sun exposure gradually. When you are tired, your metabolism is slower to react. Rest first, then take the sun!

- If your holiday is in a cooler climate, be careful not to get cold. If you do get cold, take a warm bath to warm up, and preferably then go to a warm bed to sleep for a while.

- Avoid damp. Damp (http://www.acupuncture-points.org/damp.html) can be a huge drain on your energy and makes it much harder for your Spleen energy to function properly. In your body you experience it as a sense of heaviness, soreness and even swelling eg of joints. A few days of warmth might clear it, but if it has seriously invaded your body, you will want to take painkillers either orally or locally as creams: these have their own downsides if taken for long, whereas there are 'alternative' solutions that may work just as well with few secondary effects. Some of these alternatives are explained in this book.

- Get your mind off work.

- Worry quickly drains your energy. By all means talk about it, but having done so, occupy your mind with other thoughts, perhaps by reading or gardening or meditating; or try cycling or walking with others. Get away from the source of worry! Go to a film or concert, meet friends for a meal ...

- Ongoing grief and disappointment dissipate energy. Find something to do or look forward to that helps you take your life forward. Meet considerate but cheerful friends.

- Men and their partners: to start with, less ejaculatory sex! Ejaculation uses up valuable supplies of a particular kind of energy (read much more about this at http://www.acupuncture-points.org/jing-essence.html) that you should not lose when already tired.

- Women: one cause of this (particularly for Kidney involvement) is having too many babies too closely together. Obviously this cause is not immediately remedied. It takes time! Good acupuncture would help you get stronger even when breast-feeding (herbs might make your breast milk taste odd and put your baby off breast-feeding).

- Women: if you suffer from heavy periods, see an acupuncturist or Chinese herbalist. Heavy blood loss is very draining. You need to get it fixed.

- Make sure you eat nutritious food, properly chew it, and take time to enjoy it: don't rush!

- Eat before you get tired – and do not eat large meals just before bedtime.

- Eat and drink nothing that at the time of consumption is cold, chilled or frozen. Preferably eat cooked food that is warm when you consume it.

- Eat at regular meal-times. This is a good general rule, as snacking too much between meals or towards bedtime can lead to a syndrome in Chinese medicine called *Food Retention* (http://www.acupuncture-points.org/food-retention.html ) which is more likely if you are fatigued. However, if you haven't eaten anything for some hours before bedtime, a few nuts (brazil, hazel, almond, not peanut) may help sleep.

- *Do not over-eat.* When you are tired, you have less energy for digesting food, so start with smaller meals, even if you still feel hungry afterwards. *Always chew well!*

- If a cause of your Qi deficiency is under-nourishment, consider a good nutritional supplement. Preferably use one that is made from easily digested organic vegetables and fruits, dessicated and powdered, taken with water, so reconstituting itself in your stomach before you digest it. Your body recognises foods derived from vegetables and fruit more easily than supplements made from chemicals compressed into a tablet. Fruit and vegetables contain nutrients in the right proportions for easy assimilation; tablets may not.

- Avoid junk foods, soft drinks, quick sources of energy including sugar or foods containing sugar, and processed foods; stop coffee (for why, see http://www.acupuncture-points.org/coffee.html) and other sources of caffeine; if you have a craving for chocolate or sugary foods or sweets, you may be somewhat dependent on them and may even be suffering from *candida albicans* (*thrush*) which needs professional assessment. Most of these foods deplete your supplies of Magnesium, urgently needed by enzymes in your body to promote energy production.

- If you decide to take a Magnesium supplement, find one that also contains at least Calcium, Boron, Zinc and Vitamin D which help you to absorb it. Better still, eat foods that naturally contain the mineral. Such foods usually contain fibre, such as green vegetables, legumes, bananas, avocados and nuts. However, avocados and bananas are cooling, so less suitable if you have fatigue, cold or damp phlegm.

- Every day eat a few nuts (eg walnuts, almonds, pecans, brazil, hazel) and seeds (eg sesame, sunflower, pumpkin, flax). These contain essential oils, zinc and magnesium, all of which help you recover your energy.

- Consider how to boost the natural flora of your intestines. Good food does this naturally, but fermented foods like cabbage (sauerkruat) do this fast; also dairy-based foods like yogurt, if natural and unsweetened – but diary foods may not suit everyone and, if you have read other chapters in this book, you will know that dairy foods often increase phlegm production. Acidophilus, for example, helps to maintain a healthy balance of organisms in your intestines.

- As you age, your body's metabolism deteriorates. You absorb nutrients less efficiently and may be deficient in some important minerals or vitamins. For example, as you age, you  absorb less vitamin B12, leading to anaemia, poor protein synthesis, declines in healthy cell formation and cellular longevity, all areas more or less under the aegis of your Spleen. Tests show if you need supplementation.

- Reduce alcohol or other drugs that relax you: they may relax you but your body uses its scant supplies of energy to metabolise them, i.e. to clear them out of your system.

- Not suitable for everyone, but try this. At bedtime, take a tablespoonful of organic hemp oil followed by one of olive oil. This becomes a gradual source of energy during the night and ensures that your bile duct remains clear and that your liver and gallbladder function smoothly. However, if you have just eaten a large meal before going to bed (as you will have read, further up, I do not recommend eating a large meal before bed!) there is no point loading your digestion with more, so do not take hemp and olive oil before bed on this occasion.

- Also not suitable for everyone, but try this. In the morning, take two tablespoonfuls of organic apple cider vinegar in some warm water. This stimulates your digestive system including your liver and gallbladder. It also helps your digestion, bowel movements, skin and vision.

- As you improve (sleep, rest and food come first) begin to take gentle exercise. No point trying to compete, to beat your own best: you need to learn to go slow for a while!

- Walking is an excellent way to improve your health. It makes you breathe properly and moves every artery, vein, muscle and nerve you possess.

- Poor breathing habits are bad for health in many ways: learn to breathe properly as you walk. See the advice at the end of chapter 5 just before the summary. (And don't smoke!)

- As a short-term measure, sip water infused with lemon juice. The sourness helps to reduce fluid leakage.

- *Beware infection!* You are low in energy, and more susceptible to diseases until your body recovers. You have excess mucus because you are tired, and viruses and bacteria love mucus. You are a clear target for them. Remember how important hygiene can be. Wear gloves if you touch rails or doors in public places. Use a clean handkerchief every day. Don't pick your nose. When you shake hands with someone, even someone healthy with healthy skin, their hands will carry bugs which end up on your hands, so wash your hands before eating. Basically do all those things a good mother would have taught you!

Are there herbs that help?

Choose from the following. Don't take them all at once. In fact, it is better to try them out one at a time, each for several weeks, to help you decide which suits you best. If you take several together and then feel worse, or at least no better, you will have no way to decide which to stop.

- **Ashwaganda** (*withania somnifera*) is an Indian herb that helps your body adjust and improve. Read the instructions before taking but 600 mg to 1000 mg suits many people, taken in capsule form with warm water. However, **ashwaganda is not recommended for pregnant women**.

- **American Ginseng** (*panax quinquefolis*) – which is not actually ginseng at all – is often beneficial. Take 200 mg powder twice daily with warm water. This herb works best when the weakness has occurred after a debilitating fever.

- **Cardamom** (*elettaria cardamomum*) is pungent, warm and drying, an excellent herb for use against low energy. As a Qi tonic it is not quite the same as an energy tonic, but more of a reviver of the spirit. It benefits the digestion and appetite. Part used: the fruit. How to use: buy it in the essential oil form, although by crushing the small black seeds in the fruit you can make an infusion (see appendix). As *essential oil, take 2 – 5 drops* in warm water, sipped throughout the day. Inhale the pungent vapour to help clear sinuses and behind the nose.

- Ginseng (*panax ginseng*): overuse of this herb has meant a reduction in quality and an increase in prices. The root if in good condition can be boiled many times to extract the active qualities in decoction form, and drunk as a tea. Because of quality and supply problems, I suggest you use other herbs listed here.

- **Pine needles** *(pinus sylvestris)* are pungent, with both warming, cooling, drying and moistening qualities. This is a major lung herb and excellent for Qi deficiency mucus ie fatigue phlegm. Also very good for general tiredness with a dry cough. **How to use**: *essential oil, 3-5 drops* in warm water

- **Rosemary**, *(rosemarinus officinalis)* is pungent, warming and drying, excellent for helping your body to generate warmth and to invigorate your Lungs to expel cold phlegm and to clear damp conditions from your head.   In terms of Chinese medicine it also stimulates Kidney Yang, which helps Spleen Yang and Lung Yang. It can be taken over long periods as a general warming herb, but also helps acute conditions. This is a great herb for the chest, heart and lungs, being a major yang tonic. However, that means it should not be used much, or only with caution or under guidance, if there are signs of yin deficiency (for more on yin deficiency, read http://www.acupuncture-points.org/yin-deficiency.html). **Part used**: the leaves. If from your garden, make it up as an infusion (see appendix). Otherwise, use the *essential oil: 3-4 drops* in warm water, sipped as needed. The pungent oils given off should be inhaled.

- **Sage** *(salvia officinalis)* – garden sage – is a great herb for fatigue phlegm, being dry and pungent. Recognised since antiquity for its beneficial medicinal attributes, the herb is in many ancient formulae for longevity, but it also restores the mucus membranes. If you have the herb in your garden, take 500 mls of a warm infusion (see appendix for how to make this) of the leaves, sipped throughout the day. Alternatively use the *essential oil, 2-4 drops* in warm water twice daily. **DO NOT USE SAGE if pregnant or if subject to epileptic fits**.

- **Thyme** *(thymus vulgaris)* is a common garden culinary herb, also having herbal or medicinal qualities that are often overlooked. It is pungent, warming and drying, an excellent herb for fatigue phlegm (Qi deficiency mucus). It benefits the Spleen and Lungs. **Part used:** the herb, ie the leaves. How to use: although the infusion is easy to make at home, the *essential oil* is stronger but should be taken in gelatin capsules because if the oil is swallowed, even in water, it can have a burning effect on mucous membranes. That said, a few drops in hot water make an excellent inhalant. **Warning: do not use during pregnancy**. because thyme stimulates the uterus. Also, **avoid if you are hyperthyroid**, because this herb is too yang in action for you.

- A good combination of herbs I have seen sold in shops in sachets is one containing rosemary, thyme, ashwaganda and ginseng as the main ingredients.

- A Western-style herbalist might include some of the herbs mentioned above in combination with others to help *your* particular condition.

## Chinese medicine

Please note that acupuncture and Chinese medicine can often resolve this fatigue phlegm condition within a few days.

There are Chinese herbal formulae that can greatly enhance your Qi. The most famous is **si jun zi tang**, also called the 'Four Gentleman' formula. These 'four gentlemen' are some of the most used herbs in Chinese medicine, and include ginseng. Nowadays, although ginseng is often used, it will have been artificially cultivated, and lacks the power of the wild root. It may also be contaminated with herbicides and pesticides. So there are many other formulae that do roughly the same thing, often adapted specifically to your particular needs. Most such take the basic formula, add some herbs to it and subtract others. It can be quite an art. If the formula is right for you, and assuming you discontinue the actions that caused your Qi deficiency in the first place, your energy and symptoms will normally improve within a few days.

## Summary

- Fatigue phlegm (actually increased mucus) occurs when you are tired
- *For health you need rest, good food, and sleep*
- You may need foods that are, in Chinese medicine, tonifying. These are, for almost everyone, foods/drinks with a warming quality, nearly always taken when cooked and warm
- Herbs that are warming and drying are particularly useful

*The next chapter covers **Damp** phlegm and how to deal with it.*

# Chapter 11 - Damp Phlegm and how to deal with it!

Before you speak, do you have to clear your throat? And if you stop speaking, do you find you need to swallow and hawk something up or out of the way? It can be embarrassing and awkward, and it can go on for not weeks or months, but years. This is your chapter!

Typical symptoms of *Damp Phlegm* (those most common are in **bold**) include

- **Copious sticky white phlegm** that is easy to expectorate from the lungs

- **Chest feels oppressed, a little tight or heavy**: not easy to take a satisfyingly full breath

- **Shortness of breath,** for example when taking exercise or walking uphill or upstairs

- **Chronic cough,** often brought on by eating too much, or the 'wrong' foods, or in damp environments, with spasms which produce lots of the phlegm listed above

- **Cough sounds full of phlegm**

- Wheezing leads to coughing; cough starts with a wheeze
- Upper abdomen can feel blocked or full
- Phlegm felt in the throat
- **Frequent need to clear the throat** or before speaking
- Frequently, a feeling of nausea
- Head feels muzzy and can be dizzy
- Frequent tiredness and fatigue
- Need to rest or sleep mid-afternoon
- Is worse when lying down flat: needs to lie with upper body and head raised
- **Not thirsty**
- Face Complexion is white and pasty
- **Tongue is swollen** in the middle or towards the front
- **Tongue coating is sticky and white**
- Pulse is described as '**slippery**' (but only a trained acupuncturist would be able to diagnose this)

**Damp phlegm** and **cold phlegm** have some similar qualities, which is why some of this chapter will seem similar to the chapter on cold phlegm.

But with damp phlegm there is a different emphasis. As you would expect, cold is not the problem, but *damp*, both cold and hot, and anyone who has lived in monsoon climates will know what the effect of warm damp – humidity – can be.

If you have damp phlegm, some of the following may apply:

- You got damp. This could have been through your skin, as by sitting for too long on damp grass, or by being soaked in a rainstorm and unable to get warm and dry quickly afterwards, or not drying off properly after swimming, or by being frequently exhausted in hot, damp – humid – conditions. This could have happened some time ago. Although one such occasion might be enough to bring on symptoms, usually damp enters after repeated exposure, unless some of the following also apply:

- You live, work or lived for a while in a damp place, such as a room with damp or wet walls, possibly from what is called 'rising'-damp, or caused by damp in the environment, such as a kitchen or sauna-type room, or perhaps working in wet fields or muddy conditions, especially if tired or unable to warm up properly after work. Working beside an indoors swimming pool is a potential cause of damp too.

- Living aboard a boat on the sea can promote damp if your cabin, to preserve warmth, is damp.

- The same goes for living in a caravan with closed windows, especially if cooking with gas (which in burning creates water in the air), or in a tent that never dries out. Circulate fresh air regularly through your living area.

- Dampness invading your body through your skin also produces other symptoms like heaviness and dull aching muscles; in the joints it causes swelling; in the urogenital organs it causes vaginal discharges and urinary discomfort; it sometimes culminates in vesicles on the skin: eventually it upsets the Spleen (http://www.acupuncture-points.org/spleen.html) and your digestion. All these make you more susceptible to damp phlegm in your lungs and head.

- *Over*eating – even of good foods – weakens your Spleen, Stomach, and digestion. This leads to what is called an 'accumulation' of Damp and Phlegm. For more on this see below and Spleen – http://www.acupuncture-points.org/spleen-damp-cold.html.

- *Dietary mistakes* in general cause weakness in your digestion and Spleen. The most frequent problems are a surfeit of sweet food and sugar, and foods that easily become sugars in the blood, including foods made from refined flour, or foods that have had their skins removed, such as potato crisps and chips. This also includes sweet fruits like bananas. Too many such 'sweet' foods disturb the Spleen function, leading to abdominal distension and fullness after eating, mucus in the stools, discharges from the vagina: and also mucus in the Lungs, throat, sinuses and nose – which thickens to form damp phlegm!

- *Too many 'greasy' foods* – though not all are greasy to the touch. These include **milk** and **dairy products** including cheese, yogurt, butter, cream, creme fraiche, kefir, lassi and ice-cream. This category also includes **deep-fried foods**, chips, battered foods, peanuts (especially roast peanuts) and very fatty meats, such as pork. It is the experience of people practising Chinese medicine that too many such foods lead in susceptible individuals to the formation of phlegm, manifesting in the nose and sinuses as discharges, and in the forehead as a dull headache, sometimes with mild dizziness, and respiratory problems including mucus and phlegm in the lungs and upper respiratory tract.

- *Eating too many foods with a* **Cold** *or* **Damp** *quality.* These include fruit, especially out of season or in cold or damp conditions, and foods of a *raw or cold* quality (http://www.acupuncture-points.org/cold-foods.html), including salads made with raw vegetables. Your Spleen dislikes food that is too moist or cold, including excess cold or chilled fluids. Modern Western thinking currently often favours raw fruit and salads as being full of naturally occurring vitamins and enzymes, but if your Spleen tends to be weak, digesting too many of these (uncooked or raw) foods will be difficult. Consequently you will find that your bowel movements are runny – diarrhoea, that your energy is low, that you tend to feel chilly much of the time, often have abdominal discomfort, swelling or distention after eating, possibly with flatulence, and then get increased quantities of mucus – damp phlegm!

- *Eating in poor conditions for proper digestion* and Spleen function includes eating too hurriedly, or when stressed or working or if upset; eating when tired, (say late at night); leaving no time after eating before sleeping or before returning to work. These habits deplete your Stomach energy and the proper function of your Spleen. That can lead over time to the formation of damp phlegm.

- *Malnutrition* from eating insufficiently nutritive food is a frequent cause of Spleen deficiency and the formation of Damp Phlegm. Quantity has exceeded quality: often less, but better foods properly eaten, would improve health.

- **Attacks** by what in Chinese medicine are called Wind-Heat (http://www.acupuncture-points.org/wind-heat.html and Wind-Cold (http://www.acupuncture-points.org/wind-cold.html) affect firstly your Lungs which try to defend you. If your Lungs fail to disperse the invading force, you get well-known common 'Cold' symptoms such as sneezing, chills, aches, dislike of cold, headaches, blocked nose, cough and copious discharges. Normally these clear as your body sheds the cold. If catarrh seems to remain indefinitely, you have damp or cold phlegm! Or both.

- **Worry and anxiety** over a long period weaken your Spleen so it more easily succumbs to phlegm formation.

- *Grief, disappointment, loss of close friends and family, and sadness* deplete your Lung energy. Together these can often lead to poor posture, stooping ( a sign of yang deficiency) which impedes natural lung function. Poor Lung function means that they cannot disperse accumulated fluids nor send them down to the kidneys and bladder for excretion. So these fluids hang around in the upper part of your body and respiratory tract creating damp phlegm.

- *Poor breathing patterns over a long period weaken the Lungs* and your body generally. Sedentary work, lack of exercise, often sitting (even if not stooped) at a desk for long periods does this too. For health your body needs some physical work to keep itself in order. Most important of all is regular out-of-breath chest respiration from physical activity, though deep abdominal breathing is also good. (Your lungs are the only organ which most people can control: you can decide to breathe fast or slow, or to hold your breath, whereas unless you have trained yourself you cannot speed up your pulse mentally, or increase the rate at which your liver metabolises alcohol, or that your kidneys filter blood to make urine.) Pumping breath keeps your lungs in good condition, able to disperse fluids and to keep energy flowing round your body. (This is deeper stuff than you may realise! Read more at http://www.acupuncture-points.org/lung-qi.html.) *Not* letting your lungs do their job encourages the accumulation of phlegm, which is said to be *created* by your Spleen but *stored* in your lungs.

- *Excessive physical work, or over-lifting,* or doing too many things at once or in quick rotation over a long period, or working physically for long hours for many years without proper rest, can all weaken proper functioning of Spleen Yang (http://www.acupuncture-points.org/spleen-yang.html) and Kidney Yang (http://www.acupuncture-points.org/kidney-yang-deficiency.html). Weak Yang cannot warm you up sufficiently to burn off or dry up fluids in your body. That leads to the formation of damp phlegm. Some athletes and bodybuilders, for example, always have mucus and damp phlegm because of this.

- *Voice over-use.* Some professions lead to weak Lungs because they require continued use of the voice. Teachers, actors, traders and negotiators may suffer from this. With weak Lungs you become more susceptible to damp and phlegm formation as your weakened Lungs cannot disperse and descend fluids for excretion.

- Atmospheric pollutants including from diesel fuel have increased hugely over the last 50 years, during which time we have seen a massive increase in respiratory problems. Many of these pollutants are heating in effect, creating a range of symptoms from over-sensitivity to them. When inflammation occurs in your body, it responds with extra mucus which easily becomes damp phlegm.

- Immunisation is a boon and has saved many lives. But bear in mind that immunisation pumps small but powerful fluids into your body. There are very few, if any, prospective randomised double-blind placebo-controlled trials of them. Any extra fluids pumped into you can lead to fluid accumulation and potentially phlegm.

**What to do?!**

Damp is insidious and sometimes hard to shift. (Read more about it at http://www.acupuncture-points.org/damp.html.)

However, it is important to clear damp from your body because its continued presence leads on to many other, more serious, conditions of disease. Lots of problems start with a little damp that wasn't cleared and eventually entered other places, like your joints (as in swollen or painful) or your intestines (sounds of water sloshing around, diarrhoea), your urogenital system (cystitis and discharges) or your lungs (bronchitis, bronchiectasis) and much more.

Some of the following should be obvious if you've read the list above about the causes of damp. Quite a lot of it requires a change in something you do, not just once, but ongoing. Sometimes, one small change is all that is needed.

As you change your diet and eating habits you may notice not just *less damp-phlegm* but *improved health overall:* likewise for better breathing habits.

And making some of these changes requires application. Amazingly, you may find that eating fresh food, cooked, makes you not just healthier, but less poor! Buying fresh food and cooking it is cheaper than buying ready-made food. (Cooking takes time, however – but you may find you enjoy it!)

The following list is roughly in order of importance. So the first ones listed are more important – for most people!

- **Breathing**. To do *anything* your body needs energy, and the most important energy of all comes from the air you breathe – oxygen. If your breathing is always shallow, never challenged, you will lack this vital ingredient in your blood, and your lungs and heart will grow lazy. Lazy people don't put out their garbage. Guess where your body stores its equivalent? Firstly, often in your lungs as *damp and phlegm*; secondly, in your flesh as **fat**. In either case, your body will be unable to function properly, to ward of minor diseases, to run for a bus, to care for children without exhaustion.

- Almost any physical activity that gets you out of breath will do! Walking is great! – but not window-shopping, it's too slow. You need to get out of breath for at least 15 minutes, preferably several times a day, so walk *fast*. Take up skipping or walking uphill, or climbing stairs – you are blessed if you live upstairs because instead of taking the lift, you can walk up; same on the escalator to work! For others vigorous swimming does it, but dry off quickly afterwards and get dressed: don't loll around in your bathing costume in a damp area, though a warm dry beach is usually fine if the air dries you quickly. Those whose job is physical can worry less, but for many of us proper breathing is first on this list for a good reason. *NB If you are unused to physical activity, work up to this gradually and if in doubt, seek medical advice first.*

- Read the books on breathing mentioned at the end of chapter 5, or take lessons in yoga pranayama.

- Once you breathe better, you may be surprised by what comes up as your lungs start to work again, but persevere. Once they've spring-cleaned themselves, you'll feel ridiculously better. (As for smokers/e-vapers? Stop! Have you really thought about what you are putting in your body?)

- **Improve what you eat and how you eat it.** Bad food, or food eaten badly, over-strains your digestion. Result? Tiredness, frequent fatigue; damp, later phlegm. By eating food badly, I mean rushing it, not chewing it, eating at irregular hours, eating when working or worrying, not giving your body time to digest before returning to work and so on. Read more at http://www.acupuncture-points.org/nutrition.html. As for bad food? Low-quality food leads to malnutrition, however much of it you eat.

- **Avoid living or working in damp places**. If you cannot avoid damp, make sure you dress in dry clothes, that you have plenty of fresh air circulating, that you get out into drier air regularly to breathe and exercise.

- **Do not eat sweet foods, or foods that become sweet on chewing.** These include sweeteners, wheat, bread, biscuits, cakes, sweets, sugary foods and drinks, potato, crisps, snacks etc – but observe your body to work out which of these, or other foods, are your own particular problem. *Such sweet foods are the main cause of damp. Many cold foods also increase damp, see below.*

- **Don't eat foods with a cold quality**. For Chinese medicine to work, patients are always advised to eat (good) food that has been cooked and is *eaten while still warm*. Avoid food that is raw, cold, chilled, iced or frozen (see the link for this below). That includes salads, supposedly health-giving and good-for-you, because they are cold and raw. (Which is not to tell you never to eat them if you are well, it's summer and you're feeling comfortably warm and relaxed!)

- Some foods are said to dry damp. These include *grains* such as barley, basmati rice, corn, rye; *vegetables* such as alfalfa sprouts, asparagus, button mushroom, caper, celery, corn, pumpkin, radish, turnip, parsley, daikon radish, white fungus, kohlrabi, (cooked) onion, mustard leaf, pumpkin, scallion; *fruit* such as papaya, lemon, umeboshi plum and *beans* such as aduki, lentils, kidney. Others include blue-green micro-algae, white pepper, vinegar. But make no assumptions! Try them by all means, but not all work for everyone. *See which work for you (and take them warm!)*

- **Keep dry and warm**

- Raise the head of your bed by 6 inches: this may help your body to drain phlegm from your head at night.

- **Chew food well** before swallowing

- **Avoid Cold foods** (http://www.acupuncture-points.org/cold-foods.html). These include bananas and avocados, indeed most fruit.

- Don't live or work in contact with damp cold conditions and don't sit on wet grass (just an example of where not to sit!).

- Cover up well when outside if it is cold.

- Introduce some *raw ginger root* into your diet, for instance in stir-fried dishes or stews or soups. Make a drink by putting a

slice of ginger in a mug and pouring boiled water over it –
then let it steep for a few minutes before sipping it.

- When possible, apply heat to your stomach/abdomen or
chest, such as by using a wheat-bag, or hot water bottle.

- As your body recovers, the dampness will dry. That can leave
the inside of our nose feeling dry, for a day or two and until
your Lungs put normal moist mucus back there. That
dryness can be uncomfortable, even itchy. You will find
yourself scratching or picking the inside of your nose. Try to
resist! Carry extra clean tissues or clean handkerchiefs. If you
must, use them to remove any dry caking in your nose. Don't
pick your nose with bare fingers (see "beware infection"
below, for why.). There is another argument too: by
suppressing the drying action in your nose, you potentially
suppress your body's *best* attempt at dealing with the damp
phlegm. You make it fall back on its *second best* strategy,
which is to keep the dampness inside you. That takes longer
to cure than sticking it out to dry in the wind, in your nose!

- *Beware infection!* You are low in energy, and more
susceptible to diseases until your body recovers. You have
damp phlegm because your Spleen is weakened, and viruses
and bacteria love phlegm. You are a clear target for them.
Remember how important hygiene can be. Wear gloves if
you touch rails or doors in public places. Use a clean
handkerchief every day. Don't pick your nose. Even your
keyboard carries bugs, some of them old and, if you eat at
your desk, kept in good condition by the morsels you drop
as you eat: those bugs could return to bite you! When you
shake hands with someone, even someone healthy with
healthy skin, their hands will carry bugs which end up on
your hands, so *wash your hands before eating*. Basically do all
those things a good mother would have taught you!

In addition, the following herbs may help your body overcome damp phlegm by warming you and strengthening the metabolic processes that help you expel it.

In Chinese medicine the herbs are said to 'resolve' phlegm and damp, and restore the descending function of your Lungs.

1.  The first ('resolve' phlegm and damp) stimulates your Spleen into more activity,
2.  The second ('restore the descending function') gets your Lungs working. But if you ignore the general advice above about your diet and food, you'll halt the benefits for your Spleen, and if you don't start exercising and standing properly so you can breathe better, you'll jigger your Lungs, so they won't do their job either!

Herbs in **Bold** are particularly important, and usually easy to obtain in essential oil form or to prepare yourself.

*   Aniseed *(pimpinella anisum)* is pungent, warm and dry. The pungency benefits your Lungs, and dampness is driven out by the herb's warm, dry qualities. Best form to take it is the *essential oil;* 2 – 4 drops in warm water, inhaled and sipped.

*   Angelica *(angelica archangelica)*, also pungent and drying, is even more warming than aniseed. It is also a Qi tonic. **Essential oil**, 2 – 4 drops in warm water, sipped.

*   Basil *(ocimum basilicum)* is also pungent, warm and dry. Its energy is more pure yang than drying, but the herb is still effective against damp and phlegm. *Essential oil* 2 – 5 drops in warm water.

*   **Cardamom** *(elettaria cardamomum)* is pungent, warming and drying. It benefits energy and qi, and warms and stimulates the digestion, drying out mucus damp. *Essential oil*, 2-5 drops in warm water, regularly.

- Elder flower *(sambucus nigra)* is revered in herbal folklore for its ability to clear the early stages of infections (called Wind-Heat or Wind-Cold in Chinese medicine). It is pungent and drying, but has, if anything a cooling effect. So Elderflower is probably at its best against damp when there is also Heat, helping to clear runny noses and to slow a 'cold' in its early stages. Make a hot infusion (see appendix) and sip it. If your damp phlegm remains long after the acute infection has departed, this herb may help, but you have passed the moment when it can help most.

- Fennel *(foeniculum vulgare)* is warm, drying and a little pungent. Its main action is on the urinary organs, but does warm the Lungs and Spleen to expel damp-phlegm. *Essential oil*: 1-5 drops, in warm water, sipped between meals. **Caution: do not take the essential oil if pregnant as it stimulates the uterus.**

- **Ginger** *(gingiber officinalis)* is a warming, dry, pungent herb. It benefits the digestion and the lungs. In Chinese herbal medicine it has been used traditionally to enhance absorption of other herbs in a formula, by protecting and warming the Stomach and Spleen. Being a warming herb, it is very good at helping to clear damp-phlegm and cold-phlegm conditions (NOT so good for hot-phlegm or dry-phlegm!) **Part used**: the root. Wash it but do not remove the skin. Once dried, the root may be wrapped in cling-film and kept refrigerated. (NB avoid the dried powder, often sold for culinary purposes, which is much more heating.) **How to use**: a simple decoction is made by taking a thin slice of the root, placing in a mug and pouring boiling water over it. Leave to steep until cool enough to sip. Sip three or more times a day. *The essential oil* is another convenient way to take it. 1 – 3 drops in warm water, three or more times a day, sipped. NB: ginger is a hot herb. If you suffer from ulcers (eg stomach or peptic), or other signs of heat, seek advice before taking large quantities of ginger. If you are diagnosed as having conditions known as Stomach Fire, or Lung Heat, including Lung Deficient Yin-type Heat, best to avoid it, at least as a single herb. (A trained herbalist might well safely incorporate it in a formula for these syndromes, however.)

- Hyssop *(hyssopus officinalis)* is pungent and drying, perfect for damp-phlegm and cold-phlegm conditions. It warms and relaxes the chest, lungs and bronchi. This means it helps your lungs work better and enables your body to develop the energy to breathe more deeply and to cough up or expectorate damp or cold-type phlegm. Longer-term it can help asthmatics suffering from Lung Qi deficiency, and because it also benefits the Spleen, it helps to warm your digestion and reduce phlegm formation. **The part used** is the herb, but the best way to obtain Hyssop is via the *essential oil*, 2 – 3 drops of which should be sipped in warm water several times a day. **Warning**: this is quite a strong herb and contains a camphene oil that can be toxic, especially in essential oil form, so do not exceed 3 drops as explained. Do not take it for more than a month at a time, and avoid completely if you suffer from epileptic fits. Also *avoid it during pregnancy* as it can overstimulate the uterus.

- **Onion** *(allium cepa)* shares many qualities with Garlic, but is not as strong. Like garlic, onion is hot and drying, so use it for damp and cold-type phlegm. It is best taken crushed, raw, or in a little warm water. Taken that way, its pungent qualities help to disperse the phlegm more quickly. As with garlic, it can produce a burning sensation in the stomach if taken raw, in which case combining it with a slice of ginger root in warm water may make it easier to digest. Note: when cooked, onion loses its pungent qualities. Instead, its 'sweet' qualities become more effective, nourishing and strengthening. Long-term, cooked onions and shallots should be a regular part of your diet, with excellent benefits for people with cold constitutions and a tendency to damp phlegm and cold phlegm.

• **Pine needles** *(pinus sylvestris)* are pungent, with both warming, cooling, drying and moistening qualities. It is a major lung herb. This makes it one of the few herbs that can be used for both hot and cold-type phlegm, for lung dryness and lung dampness, and for Lung yin deficiency (http://www.acupuncture-points.org/lung-yin.html). It benefits Kidney Yang deficiency (http://www.acupuncture-points.org/kidney-yang-deficiency.html), which then supports Spleen Yang (http://www.acupuncture-points.org/spleen-yang.html) and Lung Yang in resolving thick phlegm, but also supports lung yin deficiency where there is a dry cough. Pine needles are good for general fatigue, dry cough, dry-type phlegm, hard and in small quantity, damp-type phlegm, with copious white phlegm. **Part used**: the needles usually, but the inner bark, buds and cones are sometimes used. **How to use**: *essential oil*, 3-5 drops in warm water. To inhale, make a decoction or tincture (see appendix); warm and inhale it.

• **Rosemary** *(rosemarinus officinalis)* is pungent, warming and drying, hence an excellent herb for helping your body to generate warmth and to invigorate your Lungs to expel cold-type phlegm and clear damp conditions from your head. ( In terms of Chinese medicine it also stimulates Kidney Yang, which enables it to benefit Spleen Yang and Lung Yang.) It can be taken over long periods as a general warming herb, but also helps acute conditions. This is a great herb for the chest, heart and lungs, being a major yang tonic. However, that means that if there are signs of yin deficiency (http://www.acupuncture-points.org/yin-deficiency.html) it should be used only with caution or under guidance. **Part used**: the leaves. If you have it growing in your garden, make it up as an infusion (see appendix). Otherwise, use the*essential oil*:  3-4 drops in warm water, sipped as needed. The pungent oils given off should be inhaled.

- **Thyme** *(thymus vulgaris)* is a common garden culinary herb, but with many herbal/medicinal qualities. It is pungent, warming and drying, an excellent herb for damp and cold-type phlegm. It benefits the stomach and lungs, the Spleen and Lungs. It can be used for both acute and chronic conditions of the lungs. **Part used**: the herb, ie the leaves. **How to use**: although the infusion is easy to make at home from sprigs of the herb, the *essential oil* is stronger but should be taken in gelatin capsules because if the oil is swallowed, even in water, it can have a burning effect on mucous membranes. That said, a few drops of the essential oil in hot water make an excellent *inhalant*. **Warning**: *do not use during pregnancy*; thyme stimulates the uterus. Also, avoid if you are hyperthyroid because this herb is too yang.

- Watercress *(nasturtium officinale)* is pungent, warm and drying – also highly nutritious! Amongst its many qualities is that it stimulates the lungs, encouraging them to clear out damp phlegm. Try to get organically grown watercress and wash it before use. If only non-organic watercress is available, make sure you wash it very thoroughly, even if it is sold to you as 'already washed'. **Part used** – the leaves of the herb. **Best way to use it?** Apart from as a food, you can *press it* to obtain the juice: take 2 teaspoons in warm water three times a day. This is a warm herb: don't take the juice for more than a week at a time without a few days break, or you may irritate the linings of your mouth or throat.

- A good combination I have seen in shops in sachets is one containing lemon and ginger as the main ingredients.

- A Western-style herbalist might include some of the herbs mentioned above in combination with others to help *your* particular condition.

## Chinese Medicine

Please note that acupuncture can often resolve Damp phlegm within a few days.

There are also effective Chinese herbal formula for it.

[Warning – the following is a bit technical!] The basic formula, centuries old, is called **er chen tang**. This formula very much treats the Spleen, on the one hand encouraging it to move fluids around better and on the other steadying or regulating the Qi. While that is the fundamental purpose of the main herbs in it, there are other herbs that dry damp, clear phlegm and descend Stomach Qi. Because it includes herbs for this important 'descending' function, the formula also helps with more extreme conditions of damp phlegm such as nausea and vomiting, dizziness and palpitations that some people get in the presence of phlegm. Of course, as the Damp Phlegm is cleared, the cough goes, because the Lungs are no longer encumbered by it.

However, most practitioners would probably adapt the formula to your particular condition which is why it pays to see an experienced practitioner. In any case, manufacturers have developed a number of variants to the basic formula to suit different diagnoses.

*The next chapter covers* **Cold** *phlegm, which often occurs with Damp phlegm, though one or other predominates.*

# Chapter 12 - Cold Phlegm and how to deal with it!

This kind of phlegm is easy to spot, and even when you get better – see below – it is all too easy to fall back: just a relaxing beer or gin and tonic will set you back *days* of improvement. The crucial factor here is COLD. So learn to be aware of what you put in your mouth!

Typical symptoms of *Cold Phlegm* (the most common symptoms are those in **bold**) include

- **Phlegm is white and watery**, may even be a bit transparent: often coughed up

- Phlegm is not usually very thick or coloured except possibly on waking after sleep

- The phlegm is often runny, from nose, sinus, throat and lungs. It has no smell, but often increases in quantity after eating or drinking cold food or after too much food, or after any chilled or iced food or liquid eg ice-cream.

- Phlegm is felt in your throat and lungs

- **Chest feels heavy, full, oppressed, cold** (you like warmth on your chest and upper back)
- **You feel cold**, with cold arms and legs, cold feet and hands
- Your **cough and phlegm are made worse if you get cold, or go into cold air or a cold draft**
- Occasional dizziness or sense of mental confusion, better for taking deep breaths
- Tired, heavy feeling; hard to move
- You may feel less hungry, possibly nauseous
- **Tongue: swollen**, pale, with a coating that is wet and white
- **Pulse: slow, slippery and deep** (though the 'slippery' might need to be diagnosed by a trained acupuncturist)

With Cold Phlegm you may also have symptoms of Damp Phlegm, chapter 11, and of Fatigue Phlegm, chapter 10.

Why do you have this? You have *cold phlegm* because of one or more of the following:

- You probably caught a bad cold, or a succession of colds or other illnesses of the 'Wind-Cold' variety (http://www.acupuncture-points.org/wind-cold.html) and have not been able to rest enough to recover properly from it/them
- you are Kidney yang deficient (http://www.acupuncture-points.org/kidney-yang-deficiency.html)
- you allowed yourself to get cold, either once badly or, more often, mildly. Perhaps you don't wear enough?
- you eat too much cold-type food including raw – uncooked, chilled, iced or unheated food – or cooked food that is cold again by the time you consume it. For a link to cold foods, see below.

- you eat too many dairy foods, including foods such as yogurt, kefir and cheese, that are supposedly 'good' for you

- you eat too much concentrated food, such as protein drinks, vitamin pills or supplements. If you are cold, therefore yang deficient, these may be harder to digest, taking more energy.

- you drink **too much** liquid – cold, or even hot such as tea: tea *(camellia sinensis),* whether Indian or Chinese has a mildly cooling effect. (I'm not here referring to hot herbal drinks that have a *warming* effect, like ginger; tea is a herb, but its effect is diuretic and for most people ultimately mildly cooling.) The problem is not just with the *effect* of what you drink, ie cooling from tea, but the *quantity*. If you habitually carry a bottle of water and drink from it, you may be taking too much – more than your metabolism needs or can comfortably cope with.

- you don't rest enough!

- you over-exert either by lifting too much, doing too many things at once, working crazy hours or getting exhausted.

*What to do?*

1. First, consider how long it would take to heat your body up by a few degrees, even over a hot flame! Your body has got cold, which means not just in how you are feeling and your symptoms but in your ability to warm yourself up. It's that warming up function that is important. Your system has become less efficient, so you have signs of Cold. Consider an analogy: you sit in your car, cold on a cold day. Now start the engine. Unless the engine is so powerful that it can power an electric heater, you will have to wait until the engine warms up enough to heat the air that it pumps into where you sit. That may take many minutes. Your body is cold because your engine – your

metabolism – is cold AND it is working below par, even when it has warmed up. To get your engine back to normal takes a while, which is why your best choice is to seek treatment, for example from an acupuncturist or herbalist who understands these things. Meantime, here's what you can do ...

2. Realise that one dose of one of the herbs listed below won't be enough! You're going to have to organise yourself differently and keep doing so for a while:

3. Keep warm, which may mean raising the ambient air temperature via central heating and ...

4. Wear more clothing every day.

5. Stop exhausting yourself through over-strenuous activity or doing too much. However, energy permitting, a quick walk daily may help your lungs and heart stay healthy.

6. Have a hot bath. Stay in it until you start perspiring, or for no more than 15 minutes, whichever comes first. On emerging, dry yourself quickly and get dressed, or go to bed. (Taking a warm bath before bed is excellent for your 'cold' type metabolism.)

7. Rest more: sleep more.

8. Go to bed earlier than usual. Make sure your bed has enough bed clothes that you don't get cold while asleep. Unless you live in an extremely cold, noisy, polluted or theft-ridden environment, keep the window open at night. You and your lungs need fresh air, not stale, used air.

9. You may find it beneficial to lie down, warm, for a while during the day, if possible to get 25 minutes doze: don't take more time than this or you may go too deeply asleep, be unable to wake quickly, and reduce your sleep quality at night.

10. Avoid food/drinks that are cold to the touch, and food/ drinks that, even if warm, have a cold quality,

see http://www.acupuncture-points.org/cold-foods.html.
These include most fruit, including bananas and avocados.

11. *Chew what you eat slowly and often before you swallow it.
    This is really important!* Chewing breaks food down into
    smaller particles, easier to digest, but also has the effect of
    warming it before you swallow.

12. Eat food which has been cooked and is still warm when
    eaten. Hot foods need less energy to digest.

13. After meals, rest for a while before returning to work. By
    rest, this might mean a gentle walk, or sitting quietly for a
    while: a short walk is best, however.

14. Eat smaller meals than usual in the evening, because you
    will be more tired than you realise by then, and digesting
    food takes energy. When tired, your digestion becomes
    less effective, meaning you end up with more phlegm!

15. Read up about and eat foods that have a warming but not
    heating quality. Find out more at http://www.acupuncture-
    points.org/hot-foods.html. These include nuts such as pine
    nuts, pistachios and walnuts, chewed well and in small
    quantities; many meats, but especially beef, bison, lamb
    and venison; seafood such as lobster, prawns, shrimps;
    oily fish such as anchovies, herring, mackerel, salmon,
    sardines, trout and tuna. However, please don't eat just
    these foods! Eat plenty of warm, cooked vegetables too.

16. Avoid raw food, even if in supposedly healthy dishes as
    salads. Raw food is cooling and takes more heat than you
    have available to digest it.

17. Cut down on liquids, especially cold liquids, and alcohol.
    *No iced or chilled drinks.* If the only liquids available are
    cold, and you cannot avoid drinking them, sip them in very
    small quantities at a time, warming them in your mouth
    before swallowing. Note: alcohol such as spirits and red
    wine are warming but they also contain sugars which
    often produce more phlegm. If you must take alcohol, take

just a single glass, not chilled, and sip it, keeping each sip in your mouth for a while until it is warmer, before you swallow it.

18. Some foods often increase the amount of phlegm in your body. They benefit you when you have dryness, but not when you have cold or damp phlegm. To find out more, read http://www.acupuncture-points.org/phlegm-after-eating.html. In particular, note the remark about *dairy foods; dairy foods include supposedly 'good' foods like yogurt, lassi, kefir and cheese.*

19. Drink only liquids that are hot. If herbal, ensure the herbs used are warming. Never take liquids cold.

20. Buy some ginger root. Slice it thin, and put several slices in a mug. Pour boiling water over them and let the mug sit until the liquid has cooled enough to sip. Sip this regularly throughout the day. (To keep the spare ginger fresh, wrap it in cling-film, placed in the refrigerator.)

21. Good foods to include are garlic, onion, horseradish and chilli. Read more about these below and in chapter 9.

22. You may find that a warm bean bag or hot water bottle on your chest or back is very comforting. Or put your back against a warm radiator – but do not burn yourself!

23. A warm shower played on your upper back will help your lungs cough and hawk up accumulated phlegm. Dress warmly afterwards.

24. As you improve, start taking short, quick walks, to get yourself out of breath and warmed up. Or take up skipping. But do not get tired doing this and wrap up well.

25. When outside, wear not just warm clothes but something on your head. You can lose a lot of heat from your head, and you NEED that heat!

26. *Beware reinfection!* You are cold, and more susceptible to Wind-Cold diseases until your body remembers how to be warm. Remember how important hygiene can be. Wear

gloves if you touch rails or doors in public places. Use a clean handkerchief every day. Don't pick your nose. Wash your hands before eating. Basically, do what a good mother would have taught you!

27. Following, below, are herbs that may help. But you must keep taking them for a while. One dose will not be enough! Whichever you choose, use it for a week at least.

Warming herbs – choose only one and try it for a week before trying another –  that help to clear cold phlegm include:

- **Aniseed** (*pimpinella anisum*) is pungent, warming and drying, perfect for treating cold phlegm in your lungs. **Use the** *essential oil*, 2-4 drops in warm water, sipped and inhaled over a period of hours. It helps your  Lungs in many ways, and can also be useful even when you have a dry cough with wheezing. It also benefits your digestion, helping your Spleen work better, so reducing how much phlegm your body produces.

- **Basil** (*ocimum basilicum*) is a pungent, sweet and warm herb with drying qualities. It is more of a Yang tonic than aniseed, so helps your body to generate warmth, although for this you would need to take it over a long period of time. It also helps your lungs clear cold phlegm. **Part used**: the herb's leaves. **How to use:** if you have basil growing in a pot or in your garden, you can make a tincture, (see appendix): use 2-4 mls (40 – 80 drops) in warm water. Inhaling an infusion can help a head cold with cold phlegm, for instance. But the *essential oil* is much more powerful. Use 2 -5 drops in warm water. Inhale and sip. Be warned that basil also stimulates the urogenital system, so you may need to urinate more – but that urination shows your body is transforming phlegm into urine!

- **Cardamom** (*elettaria cardamomum*) is pungent, warm and drying, an excellent herb for use against cold and damp type phlegm where you cough up white phlegm in large quantities. It is also a Qi tonic: not quite the same as an energy tonic, more of a reviver of the spirit, but still, it benefits the digestion and appetite. **Part used**: the fruit. **How to use**: buy it in the *essential oil* form, although by crushing the small black seeds in the fruit you can make an infusion (see appendix). As essential oil, take 2 – 5 drops in warm water, sipped throughout the day. Inhale the pungent vapour to help clear sinuses and behind the nose.

- **Elder flower** *(sambucus nigra)* is pungent and drying. It benefits your lungs. It can be used for both hot and cold phlegm conditions, and is often used at the beginning of an infection such as a cold (Wind-Heat or Wind-Cold) to cause sweating. Its secondary action is to stimulate your lungs, to help them to get rid of phlegm. **Part used**: the flower. **How to use**: make an infusion or tincture (see appendix). Or buy the *essential oil* and use 2 – 5 drops in warm water.

- **Fennel** *(foeniculum vulgare)* is a secondary herb here, but it tastes and smells great and does have, among its qualities, the ability to warm your digestion (Spleen and Stomach, in Chinese medicine), so helping to clear damp and potentially phlegm, and likewise to stimulate your Lungs. It is better for Damp than for Cold Phlegm, but can be supportive for Cold phlegm, being pungent and warming. **Part used**: fruit or root. **How to use:** the *essential oil* is best, 1-5 drops in warm water, but otherwise grind a teaspoon of the seeds in a pestle, place them in a mug and pour warm water over them. Sip the liquid between meals.

- **Ginger**, *(gingiber officinalis)* is a hot, dry, pungent herb. It benefits the digestion and the lungs. In Chinese herbal medicine it has been used traditionally to enhance absorption of other herbs in Chinese herbal formula, by protecting and warming the Stomach and Spleen. Being a warming herb, it is very good at helping to clear cold-phlegm conditions. It is much less effective on its own at dealing with hot-phlegm or dry-phlegm, which is why in Chinese herbal formulae for hot phlegm conditions it would be added mainly to balance the cold nature of other herbs which might otherwise damage the Spleen function. (If taken in short decoction form (see appendix) and in enough quantity as a Wind-Cold invasion begins, it may reduce or stop the invasion in its track.) **Part used**: the root. Wash it but do not remove the skin. Once dried, the root may be wrapped in cling-film and kept refrigerated. (NB the dried powder, often sold for culinary purposes, is much more heating and should be avoided.) **How to use**: a simple decoction is made by taking a thin slice of the root, placing in a mug and pouring boiling water over it. Leave to steep until cool enough to sip. Sip three or more times a day. However, the *essential oil* is a convenient way to take it. 1 – 3 drops in warm water, three or more times a day, sipped. NB: ginger is a hot herb. If you suffer from ulcers (eg stomach or peptic), or other signs of heat, seek advice before taking large quantities of ginger. If you are diagnosed as having conditions known as Stomach Fire, or Lung Heat, including Lung Deficient Yin-type Heat, best to avoid it, at least as a single herb. (A trained herbalist might well safely incorporate it in a formula for these syndromes, however.)

- Horseradish *(rafanus albus)* is a pungent, hot, drying herb: yang in nature. Most British think of it as similar to mustard, to be used when beef is eaten. However, the herb is much more than that. Because of its strong warming nature, it is excellent at helping your body clear out cold. This makes it a superb food/herb to stimulate the lungs and digestion (Lungs and Spleen) to dry damp conditions and to warm and expel cold-phlegm. It also stimulates the intestines and bladder, meaning that as it gets to work to clear the phlegm you may find yourself urinating vigorously – and your bowels may be stimulated too. **Part used**: the root. **How to use**: buy horseradish in the root form, not powder or sauce. The root should be fresh. Use apple cider vinegar to create an infusion, (see appendix for how), leaving it overnight. Or make it into a tincture, or squeeze to extract the juice. Alternatively, grate the fresh root.If taking the juice, take 15 – 20 drops in warm water, sipped over a few hours.If taking the grated root, use 2 – 4 g, in warm water. Tincture: 6 – 12 drops in warm water. **Caution**: horseradish is a very hot herb! Do not use if you have inflammation anywhere, or fever or feel feverish. **Do not use during pregnancy.** Do not use if your are thyroid deficient or hyper-thyroid. Stop using it if it causes perspiration or diarrhoea.

- **Hyssop** *(hyssopus officinalis)* is one of the greatest herbs to create warmth and to expel cold phlegm. It is pungent, warming and drying. It is also great in the early stages of catching a cold (invasion by wind-cold: http://www.acupuncture-points.org/wind-cold.html) because it creates so much warmth that it makes you sweat, which often weakens or kills the invading bug. It also warms and stimulates your digestion (Stomach and Spleen). **Part used**: the herb. **How to use**: If you have the herb, make an infusion or tincture (see appendix for how), and in these forms it is safe to use for long periods. In the *essential oil* form it works much faster (2-3 drops in warm water, sipped or inhaled) but should not be used for more than four weeks at a time because of mild toxicity. Caution. as it stimulates the uterus, **do not use during pregnancy**.

- **Garlic** *(allium sativa)* is a food commonly used worldwide. It is very pungent, and in herbalism is also regarded as being slightly sweet and salty. Its main quality is that it is hot and drying. That means that is supports your Yang energy and helps to generate warmth and to clear cold.That makes it excellent for clearing cold-type phlegm, but **not good for hot-type** phlegm. (Hot-type phlegm is coloured, ie yellow or green, lumpy or thick, possibly viscous like string; has a strong smell and is usually hard to expectorate. It comes with offensive breath, sore throat, nose or sinuses, and you quite probably have a fever. Your doctor will propose that you take antibiotics though this book offers alternatives. If you take it for hot-type phlegm, it will tend to concentrate and dry it even more, making it harder to clear and tending to increase your sensation of heat.) People will argue that garlic's antibacterial qualities will reduce your infection, but this may take time and you may not be clear how much this is helping your body's natural defences.Use it for cold-type phlegm! **How to take it:** remove the papery covering round the garlic clove. Crush the clove and eat it. If necessary take it with warm water or having poured hot water over it, let it soak for a while before swallowing the water and the clove. Take up to six cloves a day in acute conditions.The downside to this is that your breath will smell of garlic, but it is the pungent smelly qualities that make it most effective and quick-acting.Other problems with garlic? It is so strong that it may cause burning in your stomach. In this case, take it with warm water, as explained, or reduce the quantity or size of the garlic clove. In addition, add a thin slice of ginger to the garlic when soaking it. The ginger helps your stomach digest the garlic. Other herbs that may ease your stomach when taken with garlic include cumin and coriander.Other ways to take garlic include it in the form of garlic pearls in which the garlic is enclosed in a soluble gelatine shell: much more convenient but as the garlic concentrate was made some time beforehand and reaches your stomach without release of vapour, it is less effective, so you need more of them.

Read the instructions on the packet. Also, you may prefer not to eat gelatin, derived from animal sources.**Caution**: garlic is a HOT food. Too much of it, by overstimulating your Yang energy, may inadvertently drain or reduce your Yin energy. This means that if you are diagnosed as having yin deficiency (see http://www.acupuncture-points.org/yin-deficiency.html) or suspect you may be Blood deficiency (see http://www.acupuncture-points.org/blood.html) this herb should be used with great caution, if at all. Because your reproductive health depends so much on your Yin energy, **avoid garlic in high dose if you are trying to get pregnant, are pregnant or are breast-feeding,** or (being male) suffer from premature ejaculation or spermatorrhea. If you suffer from spontaneous bleeding, eg nosebleeds or bleeding between menses, both of which are often signs of excess Heat, avoid garlic. NB garlic will tend to make hot-type phlegm worse, so don't use it for that!Once your immediate cold phlegm problem has been solved, you may find that a lower, daily dose of garlic keeps you fit. It has many other qualities not listed here, highly beneficial for deficient yang conditions, helping immunity and purifying your blood vessels. Long-term use may even incline you to become less cold, even hot, in which case of course garlic would be counter-productive!

- **Onion** (*Allium Cepa*) shares many qualities with Garlic, but is not quite as strong. Like garlic, onion is hot and drying, so use it for cold phlegm. It is best taken crushed, raw, or in a little warm water. Taken that way, its pungent qualities help to disperse the phlegm more quickly. As with garlic, it can produce a burning sensation in the stomach if taken raw, in which case combining it with a slice of ginger root in warm water may make it easier to digest. **The same cautions** arise as with garlic. However, most onions are not as pungent or warming as garlic so the effect is also less intense on yin or fluid deficiency (http://www.acupuncture-points.org/yin-deficiency.html). Note: when cooked, onion loses its pungent qualities. Instead, its 'sweet' qualities become more evident, nourishing and strengthening. Long-term, cooked onions and shallots should be a regular part of your diet, with excellent benefits for people with cold constitutions and any tendency to cold phlegm or damp phlegm.

- Pepper *(piper nigrum)* whether black or white, is pungent and hot. It affects the stomach and large intestine more than the lungs, so does help reduce cold and damp phlegm to some extent, but it is not one of the main herbs or foods for this. Being of yang-type energy, it warms the body so if you are cold it may help reduce the tendency for cold and damp-type phlegm. As with any strong yang herb or food, too much can aggravate existing excess yang conditions, such as inflammation (eg very sore throat, bladder infection, inflamed eyes) or high blood pressure. **Part used**: the peppercorn. **How to use**: many people add ground pepper to their food both to enhance the taste but also, from the point of view of Chinese medicine, to assist the stomach to digest it by providing warmth. You can use that warmth to increase the yang energy in your body with an infusion or decoction (see appendix). For instance, grind 1gm pepper with 30 gms ground fresh root ginger into 3 cups water. Simmer until only 1 cup of concentrate remains and sip this throughout the day. This encourages your bowels to move and reduces any tendency to vomiting, at the same time as increasing yang. (Nobody is suggesting that you'll like the taste, however.)

- **Peppermint** *(mentha x piperita)* is a pungent herb, mainly warming. In herbal medicine it is used mainly to clear invasion by Wind-Cold, but it does also warm the lungs, helping them to clear cold phlegm. **Part used**: the leaf. **How

**to use**: best taken in *essential oil* form, 2 -4 drops in warm water. However, to help clear cold phlegm in the head, infuse the leaves in very hot water and inhale the steam. **Caution**: do not use for more than a week, after which take a few days break. Peppermint is a warming herb so do not use it if you suffer from hyperacidity, or hot-type phlegm, or if you suffer from yin deficiency (http://www.acupuncture-points.org/yin-deficiency.html).

- **Pine needles** *(pinus sylvestris)* are pungent, with both warming, cooling, drying and moistening qualities. It is a major lung herb. This makes it one of the few herbs that can be used for both hot and cold-type phlegm, for lung dryness and lung dampness, and for lung yin deficiency (http://www.acupuncture-points.org/lung-yin.html). It benefits Kidney Yang deficiency (http://www.acupuncture-points.org/kidney-yang-deficiency.html), which then supports Spleen Yang and Lung Yang in resolving thick phlegm, but also supports you where there is a dry cough (which could be from lung yin deficiency). Pine needles are good for general fatigue; dry cough; dry-type phlegm which is hard and in small quantity; and damp phlegm, with copious white phlegm. **Part used**: the pine needles usually but the inner bark, buds and cones are sometimes used. **How to use**: *essential oil*, 3-5 drops in warm water. Also make a decoction or tincture; warm and inhale.

- **Thyme** *(thymus vulgaris)* is a common garden culinary herb, but with many herbal/medicinal qualities. It is pungent, warming and drying, an excellent herb for cold phlegm. It benefits the stomach and lungs, the Spleen and Lungs. It can be used for both acute and chronic conditions of the lungs. **Part used**: the herb, ie the leaves. **How to use**: although the infusion is easy to make at home from the herb's sprigs, the *essential oil* is stronger but should be taken in gelatin capsules because if the oil is swallowed, even in water, it can have a burning effect on mucous membranes. That said, a few drops of the essential oil in hot water make an excellent *inhalant*. **Warning: do not use during pregnancy**; thyme stimulates the uterus. Also, avoid if you are hyperthyroid because this herb is too yang in action.

- Watercress *(nasturtium officinale)* is pungent, warming and drying, so is excellent against damp phlegm and highly supportive against cold phlegm. **Part used**: the herb's leaves. **How to use**: the freshly pressed juice is the best way: take 2 teaspoons (10ml) in warm water three times daily. **Caution:** use organically grown watercress, carefully washed before use. Do not use continuously for more than a week, after which stop for 3 days: otherwise you may irritate the linings of your mucous membranes.

- A good combination sold in sachets in shops contains mainly cinnamon, cardamon, pepper, cloves and nutmeg. though it is not advertised as being for Cold phlegm.

- A Western-style herbalist might include some of the herbs mentioned above in combination with others to help *your* particular condition.

## Chinese medicine

Finally, acupuncturists use not just acupuncture needles but herbs. One herb that is excellent for warming specific acupuncture points on the body is called moxa (http://www.acupuncture-points.org/moxibustion.html) and this helps you overcome cold phlegm.

There are also Chinese herbal formulae, developed over 2500 years, to deal with cold phlegm. One of the main such is **ling gui zhu gan tang**. [Warning – this next bit is technical!] The main herb in the formula aims to strengthen the Spleen. This automatically helps your body clear Damp – see the chapter on the Spleen. However, another herb is warming, so increasing Yang energy and thereby stimulating Qi to move better. This movement shifts and transforms the phlegm. Your practitioner would almost certainly add other herbs to enhance these actions, adapting the formula to your particular needs, or choose another formula better suited to you.

NB! As cold phlegm disappears and you begin to think you are better, *keep taking* warm foods/drinks and avoiding cold foods/drinks! For me, an iced gin and tonic (for you an iced coke or beer?) taken too soon easily sets me back a couple of days, even when all other food and drinks I take are warm. Beware!

*The next chapter covers **Hot** phlegm and how to deal with it.*

# Chapter 13 - Hot Phlegm and how to deal with it!

Are you the kind of person who feels comfortable in just a few clothes, even in cold weather? Do people think you mad when you go out on a winter's evening in a cold climate wearing just a shirt? Do you have good circulation, warm hands and feet (even without a drink inside you)?

If so, you are probably blessed with a warm constitution and this chapter is for you ( ... although other people, with colder constitutions, can also get Hot phlegm).

People with good circulation more often get Hot phlegm, but it's not much fun! Its symptoms are typically more acute than those of Damp or Cold phlegm.

Typical symptoms of *Hot* phlegm include (the *most* typical listed are in **Bold**)

- **Phlegm is yellow and sticky, may be green**

- Productive cough, worse in warm room or warm air

- Chest feels oppressed, can be an effort to breathe

- Nausea

- **Mouth feels dry**

- **Thirst, usually for cool fluids, unless you also have Damp phlegm, when usually thirstless**

- **Face is red**

- **Head can feel distended, swollen**

- Ears are more sensitive to noise

- **Restlessness,** anxiety, even palpitations

- Skin is often greasy or moist: face can look as if oiled

- **Prefer cool air**

- Taste may be bitter or sticky

- **You feel worse in warm or hot rooms, 'muggy' weather conditions, environments or climates**

- You feel worse in noisy conditions

- **You feel a little better in cool conditions**

- With this condition you may snore when normally you don't, or snore more if normally you do!

- **Tongue body is swollen** and often red in colour; almost certainly **has a crease down the middle**

- The tongue crease may have dry or sticky yellow phlegm inside it

- **Tongue coating is often yellow and sticky or greasy**

- **Pulse** is **faster** than usual (and 'slippery' but only an acupuncturist could confirm this)

You get hot phlegm because:

- Your metabolism is naturally warm and reacts to disease with heat

- You often eat food that is heating in nature (see also http://www.acupuncture-points.org/hot-foods.html)

- NB Most junk foods and pre-prepared foods, ie ready-made food dishes that you cook in the microwave – are *heating*

- You don't take enough cooling liquids

- You don't eat enough neutral or cool-nature foods

- You take too much hot type liquid, alcohol being the most common example

- You have had a recent infection, probably of the Wind-Heat variety (http://www.acupuncture-points.org/wind-heat.html)

- If you usually have warm circulation, (ie warm hands and feet) and you recently got very stressed or angry (qi stagnation in Chinese medicine) this may have contributed to your condition.

What to do!

- Drink more cooling liquids; water, for example. You'll digest it better if you drink it at room temperature, tempted though you may be to take it chilled. Water helps to dilute and cool your hot phlegm, so be prepared to urinate more.

- If you simply aren't thirsty (phlegm and damp in Chinese medicine are often seen to block the Stomach thirst need) put some ginger root slices into hot water, let it cool and drink that. The ginger root will improve your digestion and also helps it deal with any kind of phlegm. Note: ginger is a herb with warming qualities, which you might think would be counter-productive if you have hot phlegm. Don't worry! Its warming ability benefits your Stomach, not the hot phlegm. (But *do not take* ginger *powder*, often used in the kitchen, because in this form ginger **is** *heating*.)

- Eat food, well chewed, that is neutral or cool in nature,

see http://www.acupuncture-points.org/cold-foods.html. But avoid frozen or chilled foods. Eat food at room temperature or slightly warm.

- Avoid hot foods: http://www.acupuncture-points.org/hot-foods.html and phlegm-forming foods. These include dairy food, rich food, greasy and sweet food, including sweets and sweeteners, and anything hard to digest. Foods that are too heating for you while you have hot phlegm include garlic, raw onion, chilli peppers, horseradish etc. and spices used in Indian, Thai and other 'hot' recipes e.g. curry. (This may be a blow for you! I have noticed that many people with warm circulations, the kind of people who tend to get hot phlegm, like these spices in ordinary cooking.  Unfortunately, continued use in ordinary life tends to heat you up, making you more susceptible to hot phlegm. So, when your hot phlegm has gone, by all means enjoy the occasional spices, raw onion etc, but reduce the frequency: don't have them so often or so strongly!)

- Do not over-eat because this can lead to food retention (http://www.acupuncture-points.org/food-retention.html) causing more Heat.

- Avoid hot liquids, in particular liquids which have a heating effect even if cold, such as spirits and red wine. For a while avoid all alcohol.

- Breathe fresh air, purified if necessary or if you live in an area of high air-pollution.

- Keep the ambient air cool, but not so cold that you feel chilled. Sitting beside a hot fire won't help! However, a cool breeze or air from a fan has certain dangers which Chinese medicine warns about. Unlikely though it might seem, you could end up with both hot phlegm *and* an invasion of Wind-Cold (http://www.acupuncture-points.org/wind-cold.html) or another invasion of Wind-Heat (http://www.acupuncture-points.org/wind-heat.html). So by all means keep the window open, but don't let yourself become chilled.

- Salty water is particularly good for you when used as described in chapter 9, sniffed up and circulated backwards through your posterior nasal passages, then spat out.

- In bed, keep your head raised at night.

- Cool flannels on your chest, throat or face may help clear excess heat, but remove them if you start to feel cold.

- *Beware reinfection!* You are blessed with a warm constitution or you are currently suffering from a hot-type condition! But as mentioned above this makes you more susceptible to Wind-Heat type disease or even Wind-Cold diseases until your body remembers how to re-balance. Remember how important hygiene can be. Wear gloves if you touch rails or doors in public places. Use a clean handkerchief every day. Use a different towel to other people. Basically do all those things a good mother would have taught you.

- Don't pick your nose with your fingers. The hotter the phlegm, the more it dries, caking the inside of your nose, even though it may not be dry in your throat or lungs. This phlegm *caking* can obstruct easy breathing. The natural tendency is to pick your nose! It is a huge temptation, hard to resist. What to do? 1. As mentioned above, sniff up salty water to moisten and wash the stuff away by spitting it out. 2. Blow your nose gently into a clean handkerchief to clear as much of the phlegm before it dries, although this is a very temporary measure because your body will soon deposit more there. 3. If you must pick your nose, use a clean handkerchief or tissue. Do not touch your nose with your hands or fingers. Re-infection is easy, and bear in mind that until your body sorts itself out using other advice or herbs here, new deposits of phlegm will soon arrive. (There's another argument for this too: your body wants to clear its phlegm. Shunting it to your nose, the outside, is a good move. If you suppress that by picking your nose too often, you may stop your body's best attempt at dealing with it. Guess what? You push it back to its second best attempt, which is storing the phlegm inside you. Guess where? Your throat and lungs!)

• More on re-infection: every time you shake someone's hand; buy something; handle letters; pick up a shovel; type on a keyboard – even your keyboard, unused by anyone else; drive a car or open a door ..., you are putting old or new viruses and bacteria back on your skin. Those bugs just *love* hot phlegm: it is paradise for them until your body develops immunity. So be careful! Wash your hands before eating! *Observe good hygiene.*

In addition, take herbs such as the following, which help to clear heat, restrain any infection and get rid of your hot phlegm – but try them one at a time, each for a few days to see which suits you best:

• **Camomile** *(anthemis nobilis)* is a wonderfully soothing herb which, among many qualities, is both cooling and moistening. Best taken by inhalation of an infusion or of the *essential oil*, 3 drops in warm water. It is even more beneficial if Qi Stagnation (http://www.acupuncture-points.org/qi-stagnation.html) is part of your picture, meaning that a possible contributing cause to your hot phlegm has been stress, frustration or emotional tension.

• **Elder flower** *(sambuca nigra)* is a pungent herb, but one that also cools and dries. So it is excellent for hot phlegm in the lungs (pungent herbs are particularly effective for lung conditions). **Use a tincture or infusion made from the**

**flowers**, sipped in warm water. However, you can now buy Elder flower in *essential oil* form, in which case take the dose recommended on the label.

- **Eucalyptus** *(eucalyptus globulus)* is a herb with superb benefits for phlegm. Its main action is cooling and its pungency makes it very effective in clearing sinus and post-nasal passageways. Eucalyptus also has yin enhancing powers, so while this is a herb that mainly benefits hot phlegm conditions, clears stringy and difficult mucus, it also soothes the lungs. It is excellent for early stage Wind-Heat invasion (for link, see below). However, because it is so pungent, it may be painful where there is acute tissue inflammation: better wait until the inflammation has reduced somewhat. Use the*essential oil*: 2 – 5 drops in warm water, up to three times daily. Sip *and* inhale. (Note: this herb has many other excellent abilities, not least to clear toxins and promote tissue repairs. It is also good for many kinds of periodic and recurrent fevers.)

- **Melissa** *(melissa officinalis)*, also known as Balm, Lemon Balm, is a cooling, drying astringent herb, so is great for Hot phlegm. Besides this it has many other qualities, including being calming and stabilising. It is useful in the early stages of a Wind-Heat type cold or infection (http://www.acupuncture-points.org/wind-heat.html) to make you sweat it out. Use its*essential oil*, 1-2 drops in warm water, sipped.

- **Pleurisy root** *(asclepias tuberosa)*, also known as yellow milkweed or butterfly weed, is pungent, cool and drying. It is an excellent herb to clear Heat and to help your body expel hot phlegm. It is often used in chronic conditions such as asthma because it helps to release Lung energy stagnation and to stop spasms. It is an excellent expectorant. **Part used**: the root.  You can buy it as a liquid tincture – in this form take 1 – 3 ml (20 – 60 drops) in warm water three times a day. **Caution**: because pleurisy root stimulates the uterus, **avoid it if you are pregnant**.

- A good combination I've seen in health shops in sachets contains eucalyptus, licorice, ginger and mullein (a cool and moisturising herb). However, this is not advertised as being good for Hot phlegm.

- A Western-style herbalist might include some of the herbs mentioned above in combination with others to help *your* particular condition.

## Chinese medicine

A good acupuncturist can help too. There are many powerful acupuncture treatments for hot phlegm. Your acupuncturist might also give you a Chinese herbal formula – really effective.

The basic Chinese herbal formula for Hot phlegm is **wen dan tang**, originally formulated centuries ago. [This next bit is technical: be warned!] Since then the formula has evolved to deal with what is called an imbalance between Stomach and Gallbladder, with Hot Phlegm. The main purpose of the formula is to clear Heat and Phlegm from your Stomach and Gallbladder and descend 'rebellious' uprising Qi. Other herbs in the modern formula help to clear Damp and regulate or harmonise the Stomach, strengthen the Spleen and keep you calm. Be Careful! Not all over-the-counter forms of this formula are the same because often the pill manufacturers put their own slant on it. So consult someone who can accurately diagnose your particular condition and make the right prescription, or choose another formula better suited to you.

As your hot phlegm subsides, you may just possibly be left with cold phlegm or damp phlegm, although this is unlikely for naturally warm people, meaning those with very good circulation, warm hands and feet etc.. To see what to do, read up the appropriate pages.

Don't ignore cold or damp phlegm, which can hang around, reducing your energy for ages. And don't pick your nose!

*The next chapter is on Dry phlegm, which people with Hot phlegm often think they get too, although usually Dry phlegm comes another way.*

# Chapter 14 - Dry Phlegm and how to deal with it

As we age, a number of conditions encroach on our health. Dry phlegm is one of them. Because it can be so hard to expel, it can be exhausting, wearing us down at a time of life when our energy is already depleted.

**Common symptoms of dry phlegm (most typical in Bold) include:**

- **Dry cough**, worse in hot or dry air, warm rooms, in hot streams of air such as a blow heater
- **Phlegm is yellow or yellow-white, powdery or pellety or stringy, sticky and stretchy (viscid): hard to cough up**
- **Chest feels oppressed, heavy, tight, constrained: may have wheezing**
- **Inside nose feels dry**
- **Throat feels dry or with small amounts of phlegm**
- **Mouth feels dry**

- Phlegm brought up may contain blood
- Shortness of breath
- Stools are dry and hard to 'move'
- Urine is scanty and dark
- Skin is dry
- Fever is possible
- Sensation of heat in the afternoon, possibly with noises in the ears, sweating at night, backpain, restlessness and anxiety
- Head feels heavy or muzzy
- Mild dizziness
- Complexion is dry and pasty coloured
- **Tongue body is swollen**
- Tongue coating is white, thin and dry, may be sticky
- Tongue body colour: tip may be red
- Pulse: thin or fine and 'slippery' (a pulse quality that might require an acupuncturist to confirm)

You may not have all these symptoms! In fact you may only have a few of them; those in bold are the most likely, and even if you had only a dry cough and it was very difficult to expectorate any phlegm, though there was some, that would probably be enough to diagnose 'dry-phlegm' in your lungs.

## How did you get dry phlegm?

Although having hot phlegm just might lead on to having dry phlegm in place of it, it is unlikely, unless the following also applied but note that it **is** possible to have hot phlegm and dry phlegm at the same time!

- Your eating habits and the kinds of food you eat cause what Chinese medicine calls 'Heat' and 'Dryness'.

- Eating habits which might lead to dry phlegm include what are called irregular or bad dietary habits over a period of time, probably months or years, such as (take a deep breath …!) eating without regular meals, eating on the go, eating while working, eating while exercising, eating while arguing, or while rushing, eating a lot or a little because of the time available and not because of your body's needs, swallowing food without chewing it properly, eating foods that lack nutrition, adding too many additives – flavourings or spices – to food before you eat it, making up for bad food habits with nutritional supplements which your body cannot digest properly, eating when also drinking alcohol, forcing your body to perform with caffeine (which warms but eventually exhausts you), returning to work too quickly after food, sleeping too soon after food, being stressed when your body is digesting food, being over-excited or cross while eating or digesting, being unable to urinate or defecate when your body needs to. *(I could have made this into a list of bullet-points – but you'd have skipped over that too.)*

- The kinds of food that, over time, will heat and dry you, tending to produce dry phlegm include 'hot-type foods' (http://www.acupuncture-points.org/hot-foods.html) eaten without enough balance from neutral or cool type foods. The most common heating foods are those full of saturated fats; foods covered in batter; dairy foods, cheese, butter etc; red meats; preserved meats; spicy foods, pungent foods, full of peppers, chillis and curries; the frequent addition of too much garlic, hot spices like dried ginger powder, mustard, horseradish, black pepper, or chilli sauces.

- Very concentrated foods, and pre-prepared foods, fast foods, take-away foods, are often heating.

- Concentrated foods include highly refined foods, such as from white flour and sweets. They give you energy but they require energy to digest, and often you get a good feeling after eating but then a 'low' energy feeling with irritability or fatigue a bare half-hour later.

- Foods can be made hotter by roasting, barbecuing, frying, deep-frying and to a lesser extent by baking them.

- Other heating foods include hot spices, jalapeño pepper, strong alcohol, garlic, onion and ginger; some meats too, especially lamb and deer meat.

- Alcohol and other social drugs are nearly always heating, especially when taken regularly over a long time.

- You may be growing old: the elderly are much more prone to dry phlegm. Their digestions are less efficient; their teeth can't chew so well; they don't eat as many vegetables as they did; they start to prefer highly flavoured foods that are more heating; their bodies become more spare and/or less resilient to heat (see also yin deficiency, next). They drink less (because as they age they urinate more frequently) and what they do drink is likely either to heat or dehydrate them. So they become more prone to heat and dryness.

- Yin deficient people (see http://www.acupuncture-points.org/yin-deficiency.html) are also more likely to develop dry phlegm.

- You can make yourself more yin deficient by taking stimulants, such as coffee. If you are young and healthy, you won't notice much difference. As you grow older, you will find that you feel tired some hours after a strong coffee, or you get tinnitus (noises in your ears) or your ears feel blocked or hotter; you may also feel in low spirits or tired.

- Any living, warm, comparatively-static body will tend over time to dry any phlegm it contains. Dry phlegm may not appear until Spring, Summer or Autumn, during or after weather which is either warming, heating or drying, or until you move into a living space that is much warmer or drier than you are used to.

- Some forms of medication tend to make you Lung yin deficient, others produce phlegm and some are drying. Although the side or secondary effects of most medications are now listed, whatever the list says, it is how YOUR body reacts to the drug that counts. Antibiotics, for example, have a very cooling effect, weakening your Stomach's yang energy, so making it less able to digest food and more susceptible to infection passing through into your intestines. At the same time antibiotics kill the good bacteria on which you depend for health. Consequently you absorb less good nutrients and may absorb more bad nutrients, making you less resilient, which is another way of saying yin deficient.

- You may have had another kind of phlegm for many years (eg, damp, cold or hot). Over many years these can be transformed into dry phlegm.

How to deal with dry phlegm

The challenge recognised in Chinese medicine is to

- moisturise the phlegm, to make it easier to flush away, then

- resolve it (i.e. help your body clear it out), and ...

- strengthen your lungs so that they become strong enough to 'descend' the oxygen ('life') which your lungs absorb from the air down to where it is needed via the blood, and

- ensure your Lungs do not become yin deficient.

This means that

1. You must improve your diet and eating habits or your problem will recur. Avoid the wrong foods, eat the right foods and start improving your eating habits – see above. Eat slowly; chew well before swallowing.
2. You need more moisturising foods, but you should eat them cooked and warm, not cold. If you are given raw fruit, such as apples, eat them only after other warm foods, and chew them well before swallowing. Moisturising foods include vegetables and oils such as olive and coconut oil, and fish including fish oils (though too many saturated fats as from animal meats would be heating). Small amounts of fruit will help unless you tend to have poor circulation or the weather is cold.
3. More specifically, the following foods are said to clear or eliminate dryness: apple, asparagus, bananas, barley, most beans, carrots, clam, millet, mussel, peanuts (*not* roasted), pears, persimmon, pine nut, oyster, pineapple, pork and pork kidney, porridge, potato, seaweed, sesame seeds, soy (tofu, tempeh, soy milk, miso), spinach, sweet potato, sweet rice, tangerine, taro, water chestnuts, yam. These should enter your diet on a regular basis: dry phlegm takes time to clear. (**Warning** – see paragraph 4/ next below. Many of the foods listed above are sweet or slightly sweet eg bananas, carrots, pears, porridge, potato, sweet rice, etc.. When you have rid yourself of your dry phlegm, please reduce these foods in your diet. If you don't, being sweet they will tend to weaken your Spleen, leading to the formation of damp and phlegm once again.)
4. Also take honey, barley malt, sugar cane and whole sugar, but use these sweeteners medicinally i.e. only in very small doses, because too many sweeteners harm your Spleen, which responds with more phlegm! The reason for taking

them is that they are moistening, and may produce mucus or damp phlegm which helps you to clear your  dry phlegm. To repeat!:  *Medicinally* means adding them in small quantities to your diet and not as an ongoing permanent measure. Unfortunately as you age  you may increasingly crave the sweet taste so be careful! And avoid refined sugars such as white sugar, demerera sugar, icing sugar etc. Use only the unrefined forms.

5. Avoid dried and drying foods. Examples of drying foods are bread and toast, and foods that have been preserved by drying them or treating them with hot spices. If you use dried food (eg soup powder, dried seaweed) fully hydrate it before cooking. (Many processed foods are dried during manufacture. Many fruits, fish and meats are dried to preserve them.)

6. Avoid hot pungent food like chilli, garlic, pepper. They heat and dry, exactly the opposite of what you need.

7. Stop coffee, which is only temporarily stimulating and warming. Its secondary effect is to drain your yin energy. To understand this in more depth, read http://www.acupuncture-points.org/coffee.html. Any tendency to yin deficiency will increase the possibility of heat and drying, the opposite of what you need.

8. Reduce or stop alcohol and social drugs until better: these are almost always yang – warming and drying.

9. Don't smoke! It heats, dries, and leaves a carbon deposit that stops your lungs breathing properly and is a poison that we now know will probably kill you. Even smoke made to taste cooling is fooling your senses. E-vape cigarettes are too new to be certain about this but they still put smoke inside you, so are likely to be harmful, and drying.

10. Drink more water, preferably warm, with ginger slices in it. This helps your Spleen and Stomach work better. It is your Spleen that when disordered, in Chinese medicine,

ultimately makes phlegm. When your Spleen and Stomach are working well, you will have more energy, your digestion will improve, your bowels will be more regular (although this also depends on your lungs) and you will lose the phlegm.

11. *If your phlegm is not just dry but **hot**,* this is one of those few occasions when dealing with phlegm when it is all right to take dairy foods, which themselves produce phlegm but more dilute. They are often chilled (eg unsweetened and natural yogurt, ice-cream or sorbet) so very pleasantly cooling. But it is easy to overstep the mark and increase the overall amount of phlegm, so you have to be careful!

12. Start taking enough fresh air exercise to get out of breath and improve, over time, your lung function. Your lungs have a major role in balancing the fluids in your body, and mucus is one of the fluids in question. How much exercise to take? Try to get out of breath at least twice a day, preferably for at least 15 minutes each time, but work up to it. Take medical advice before starting if you are unsure.

13. Try not to sit for long periods, at a desk for example. Sitting still is like a compost heap! When you put newly cut grass onto your compost heap, it begins to cook, heating the ingredients. Likewise, if your digestion is slow and you sit still, it encourages Heat  to develop. Heat dries. To avoid this you need to stretch and bend your body, to encourage it to breathe properly. If you sit still you breathe shallowly which doesn't help your body to shift the dry phlegm. Likewise if you lie in bed to relax: even though stretched your lungs are not exercised. Every 20 minutes get up and move around – get out of breath! To begin with this is difficult if you are old and unfit, but even a little movement will help: the more you do the easier it becomes.

14. **Salty water** is particularly good for you when used as described in chapter 9, sniffed up and allowed to circulate

backwards through your posterior nasal passages, then spat out.

15. Salty water does not, however, reach the phlegm drying in your lungs. For that you need air and movement (see above) and the right moisturising inhalants – see below.

16. *Beware re-infection*. Whether from hot-type or cold-type diseases makes no difference because dryness occurs both when there is yin deficiency and when there is not enough yang energy to move and circulate fluids. So take care to wash your hands regularly and most certainly before eating. Carry clean tissues or handkerchiefs to help you remove caked deposits in your nose. Don't touch your nose or eyes with your bare skin, always use a clean tissue. Remember that every time you touch a public rail, type at your keyboard, shake hands, or exchange something physically, you collect bugs. Bugs look for weakness in you, and with uncertain yang and deficient yin you are certainly a target. *Observe good hygiene and do what a good mother would have told you to do!*

Not many easily available herbs clear dry phlegm and/or reduce Lung yin deficiency. Try each of the following in turn for a few days to see which suits you.

- **Camomile** *(anthemis nobilis)* has various qualities, one of which is that it is moist and warm, but can also be cooling so it is worth trying for dry phlegm, using the *essential oil,* 2-4 drops in a little warm water, sipped occasionally. **Caution: do not use this essential oil during pregnancy.**

- *Comfrey (symphytum officinalis)*, also called boneset, knitbone and bruisewort, is a herb with cooling, moistening qualities, and is traditionally used to strengthen yin qualities in the body – hence its use in damage to bones, for which it is well-known. I list it here only because I have seen it being recommended for phlegm. However, while it does moisten the lungs, throat and nose, it is not a strong phlegm-resolving herb. This herb, if used for respiratory conditions, is more for dry coughs, and lung-yin deficiency conditions. It is not a herb for cold-phlegm conditions and not really a main herb for hot-phlegm either. It may help with dry phlegm conditions. So, if after a long period of debilitating coughing there remains considerable lung-yin deficiency, this herb can be very useful in restoring lung function. Part used: the root and leaf. Method – decoction for the root, infusion or short decoction for the leaves. However, for lung-yin deficiency and dry coughs, use it in a syrup (see appendix). Do realise that syrup contains a high proportion of sugar and this is one of those situations where sugar is beneficial for its medicinal moisturising qualities. But if taken for too long, the sugars would eventually damage your Spleen, tending to spleen deficiency conditions which, as explained earlier, do indeed lead to phlegm formation. Note: comfrey if taken in high quantities for too long is considered in some countries to be toxic. No doubt the same would apply to Marmite and Vegemite.

- **Eucalyptus** *(eucalyptus globulus)* is a herb with superb benefits for phlegm. Although its main action is cooling, its pungency makes it very effective in clearing sinus and post-nasal passageways. Eucalyptus also has yin enhancing powers, so this is a herb that mainly benefits hot and dry phlegm conditions, clears stringy, difficult mucus and soothes the lungs. It is also excellent for early stage Wind-Heat invasion (http://www.acupuncture-points.org/wind-heat.html). However, because it is so pungent, it may be painful where there is acute tissue inflammation: better wait until the inflammation has reduced somewhat. How to use. Use the *essential oil:* 2 – 5 drops in warm water, up to three times daily. Sip and inhale. Note: this herb has many other excellent abilities, not least to clear toxin and promote tissue repair but also for many kinds of recurrent fevers.

- Mullein *(verbascum thapsiforme)* is cool and moistening: a yin tonic. It is therefore mainly for hot phlegm and dry phlegm where the cough is dry, possibly hacking, with only small quantities of phlegm, hard to expel. Part used: the leaf and the flower. How to use: short decoction (see appendix). Note: if drunk hot, mullein causes perspiration.

- Pleurisy root *(Asclepias tuberosa)*, also known as yellow milkweed or butterfly weed, is pungent, cool and de-congesting though a little drying. It is an excellent herb to clear Heat and to help your body expel hot phlegm so has also been used for Dry phlegm. It is often used in chronic conditions such as asthma because it helps to release Lung energy and stop spasms. It is an excellent expectorant. Part used: the root. How to use: in decoction, but the tincture is more Lung strengthening. In tincture form, take 1 – 3 ml in warm water. **Caution: because pleurisy root stimulates the uterus, avoid if pregnant.**

- A good combination I've seen in health shops has sachets containing apple and ginger. Apple is cool and moistening, and ginger helps the Spleen work better. Another combination contains camomile, vanilla, mullein and honey. Avoid lemon and ginger, however, as this is too astringent and drying.

- A Western-style herbalist might include some of the herbs mentioned above in combination with others to help *your* particular condition.

## Chinese medicine

As it understands the roots of Dry phlegm and has a strategy for dealing with it, do consider acupuncture for treatment. However, Dry phlegm in the elderly can take a while to clear.

There are also Chinese Herbal formulae which have been developed precisely for this.

The basic formula, centuries old, is **bei mu gua lou tang.** [Warning! The following is a bit technical!] The main purpose of the formula is to moisten the Lungs and cool or clear the Heat, because that is what is drying the fluids into phlegm. Secondly, it transforms the phlegm/fluids, which enables you to urinate them out. Other herbs encourage the Spleen to perform better, transforming unwanted fluids and transporting them away. Practitioners would adapt the formula to your particular diagnosis or choose another formula better suited to you.

*The next chapter takes us into darker territory. The concept of Phlegm in Chinese medicine underlies many serious diseases, some of them fatal. You should not treat yourself with the methods outlined so far in this book if you have one of the conditions described next. Seek professional advice.*

# Chapter 15 - Other kinds of phlegm - Serious Stuff!

The concept of phlegm goes much further than the yucky stuff you've read about so far, the so-called '*substantial*' phlegm.

This chapter is about what in Chinese medicine is called '*non-substantial*' phlegm. The theory for non-substantial phlegm and its consequences goes much deeper than for 'substantial' phlegm: non-substantial phlegm is a base for potentially serious, even life-threatening disease.

This chapter, which is really just for information, explains some of the ways that non-substantial phlegm manifests, but not what to do about them. You need to see a professional practitioner for that.

Phlegm in Chinese medicine is a big complicated subject. It accompanies many syndromes and is often suspected even where it is not visibly self-evident – *non-substantial*.

When someone has a chronic condition, Yin and Yang will be out of balance; one of them will predominate eventually leading to too much or too little fluid. Either way stops the natural fluids of the body moving around as they should.

Why does having too much or too little fluid cause a problem? Think of a river, flowing naturally. People can row or sail up and down it, its moisture nourishes the fields in the vicinity and it powers pumps and dams.

- Then think what happens when there is too much water, possibly dammed up by a blockage downstream. Here it may overflow, blocking the fields and roads; bridges once easily navigated are now too low to take your boat underneath and river traffic is impeded.

- Too little water, and you can see the river bed containing just puddles.  The water lacks force and direction and is useless for navigation.

For example, too much fluid (excess Yin) acts as a brake and

- if it impedes the natural ascending and descending functions of the Lungs, fluid – phlegm – can collect in the lungs causing difficulty breathing, with excess fluids causing cough

- If as phlegm it prevents natural movement between yin and yang, the Heart and the Kidneys will stop working together, leading to mental instability or aberrations, anxiety, insomnia, lumbar pain, restlessness and palpitations; sometimes coldness too

- if it forms phlegm in the Stomach, it leads to too much 'fluid' there, causing thirstlessness, nausea or vomiting, or the feeling of a lump; also a feeling of fullness in the upper abdomen, or tightness under the ribs

- If phlegm collects in the lower abdomen, it may lead to loose stools, diarrhoea, urinary problems

- if phlegm blockage below (yin not functioning properly) leads to Qi ascending to the head (yang excess above, unrestrained by yin below), you may get dizziness, lightheadedness or a sense of 'spaciness' and headaches

- Phlegm in the lower abdomen may be partly responsible for

women having irregular periods, leukorrhoea, abdominal masses and even infertility

- If it impedes the natural flow of Qi along an acupuncture channel, you may begin to see small soft masses or swellings under the skin: 'fat nodes'

- If it blocks the natural flow of Qi in the channels nourishing the nerves and other tissues, it may also cause pain, tingling or numbness

A well-known saying in Chinese medicine is that instead of concentrating on phlegm to treat it, one should make sure Qi is moving smoothly. When Qi moves smoothly, phlegm moves on. Hence the importance of not doing anything to halt or slow the natural movement of Qi. That means putting yin and yang into balance by working to clear the causes of any Qi stagnation.

But there is another reason why phlegm can collect: deficient Yin – too little of the cooling, moisturising Yin form of Qi. This leads to a kind of dry or hot phlegm that continues often into old age. No amount of antibiotics will cure it. Like those puddles in the river bed, nothing can flow.

So, *non-substantial* forms of phlegm can manifest physically:

- Under the skin. Swollen lymph nodes and nerve ganglia, lipomas and thyroid gland swellings, breast lumps, soft palpable masses wherever occurring can all be diagnosed as what is called non-substantial phlegm. You can usually actually see these swellings, but the phlegm in them cannot be touched directly.

- Qi-type phlegm occurs where, because of qi stagnation (http://www.acupuncture-points.org/qi-stagnation.html) you feel a frog or lump in your throat; the Chinese call it a 'plum-stone'. This happens when you are angry, embarrassed or depressed, and goes when the mood clears. It is caused by Qi getting blocked by your 'unpleasant' emotions. There is a saying in Chinese medicine that phlegm goes where Qi goes, so if Qi gets blocked, phlegm gets stuck there. However, with plum-stone qi-phlegm, there is no actual phlegm, although it feels like it. Treatment with acupuncture is usually to move the qi and help you deal with your emotional reactions. The treatment is usually very successful.

- In your joints. When joints become distorted, for example from rheumatoid arthritis, the swelling is deemed to be because your body has been unable to resolve phlegm, often because of inflammation, which dries the phlegm, eventually hardening it into deformed bone. By this stage the hardened 'phlegm' has become very difficult to clear, although the stiffness and pain are often highly susceptible to acupuncture.

- In the limbs. This comes with a general heavy weariness, muscular pain, thirstlessness, copious white expectoration from cough, inability to perspire and a swollen tongue with a adhesive white coat. In many ways this pattern has some similarity with that seen in fibromyalgia and the general syndrome of 'damp' (http://www.acupuncture-points.org/damp.html).

- In your abdomen, which with this form of non-substantial phlegm feels full and swollen as if fluids are rolling around inside you; occasional vomiting of watery fluids; no thirst in spite of a dry mouth.

- When phlegm stops clear yang from ascending to the head, or gets trapped there from a history of yang excess, it causes dizziness, muzziness, mental confusion, poor concentration, severe depression, even paranoia. It can also lead to hyperactivity and obsessive traits.

- On your skin, phlegm can occur with ulcers and exudations

of sticky phlegmy stuff; sores fail to heal, or the skin thickens much more than usual and remains thick.

- Sometimes phlegm blockages cause palpitations, anxiety, insomnia, with physical problems such as fainting or convulsions, and can amount to mental disturbance.

- Stones in the gallbladder or kidneys are considered to be 'dried' phlegm, formed from fluids that have been heated and concentrated from Heat over a considerable period of time. This Heat comes from imbalanced metabolic processes in your body. (See http://www.acupuncture-points.org/Heat.html)

- Along your acupuncture channels. This occurs mostly in older people when they get numbness along their arms and legs. It is sometimes a warning sign of impending stroke, or one of its sequellae. In another form ...

- In pains, eg headache, where phlegm stops Qi from moving along the channels, pain can be felt in small spots, sensitive to touch

- Being obese – overweight – displays signs of phlegm.

- Non-substantial phlegm is also often a cause of cancer (the phlegm is said to have formed into lumps, possibly caused by a history of Qi stagnation, or of lack of physical movement), heart disease (when phlegm, sometimes suppressed by drugs, goes inwards to the chest and blocks the heart energy) or stroke (phlegm blocks the ascending/descending functions of yin and yang, so that yang, often from extreme Heat or Qi stagnation and no longer anchored by yin, cannot be prevented from rushing up to the head).

Another form of phlegm appears mentally:

- In what is said to be your 'Heart' – what most Westerners call the 'Mind' – it may lead to mental states like epilepsy, manic depression and schizophrenia.

- In a milder form it can cause dizziness, confusion, anxiety, heavy tiredness and depression, often seen in dementia. What that means is that some forms of dementia might be successfully treated with Chinese medicine (for example, herbal formulae or acupuncture) if phlegm were the syndrome diagnosed. The syndrome of 'phlegm' would have to be refined further, for instance into cold-phlegm, hot-phlegm etc. in order to apply the correct treatment.

You will understand from these examples that phlegm is an important concept in Chinese medicine, and can be not just a result of many conditions but itself responsible for many serious diseases. Phlegm diseases can be complicated to diagnose and treat. Please do not try to treat yourself!

All the more important, then, to set up and maintain the right health habits for your body!

# Chapter 16 - Conclusion

So, to clear your phlegm in the short term you need to know what kind it is:

- fatigue
- damp
- cold
- hot or
- dry

Then you need to apply the correct habits and herbs.
To clear phlegm long-term, you need to understand how

- your digestion is absolutely crucial – Spleen and Stomach
- your Lungs move phlegm and send it down to your Kidneys
- your Kidneys filter it, sending clear moisture upwards to your lungs, and helping you to excrete the rest
- your emotions can play a huge part in preventing your body from clearing its phlegm

That's about it for the simpler forms of phlegm. What can go wrong? What kinds of complications could there be?

## Complicating factors

Lots! For example if an external pathogenic factor (http://www.acupuncture-points.org/external-causes-of-disease.html) – such as a bug/bacteria/virus – is Hot and is blocking the Lung Qi from disseminating fluids, you get a thick, sticky or green phlegm that is often smelly.

If the invading pathogen has produced a Cold reaction, then the phlegm is clear, more runny and odourless.

In both cases, the body may clear the invader but be unable to clear the Phlegm. Sometimes the invader appears to remain. During treatment, symptoms of the original invasion may then return before the body can eliminate both invader and Phlegm. The temptation to suppress it again with painkillers is hard to resist, but it is often better to let it run its course, particularly in young or otherwise healthy people with good vitality. Suppressing it again may weaken the body even more, making it more susceptible to a return of the chronic phlegm.

Sometimes the patient gets repeated attacks of what seems to be Wind-Cold (http://www.acupuncture-points.org/wind-cold.html) when actually it is not a deficient immune system but Phlegm blocking the 'qi passageways' and preventing your immune force from being circulated to the exterior. In this case, trying to strengthen your immune force wouldn't work until the Phlegm had been cleared.

A further problem is that once Phlegm gets into the system, especially if that of an older, weaker person with a system which can't clear it, it becomes self-perpetuating and slows everything down, causing more fluids to stagnate leading to more Phlegm.

This is common where someone eats a poor diet, not

recognising which foods to avoid. Dairy foods are often better avoided if you have Phlegm.

Western medically trained doctors, not trained in energetic-type medicine, typically use medications that prevent the body making the long-term repairs needed. (For more about primary and secondary effects, see http://www.acupuncture-points.org/primary-and-secondary-actions.html.)

For instance

- In the case of hot or dry phlegm, hot-dry bronchodilators may make symptoms temporarily better (cooling) but then worse (drying and warming).

- Where there is blockage or what seems like an inflammation from Yin deficiency (http://www.acupuncture-points.org/yin-deficiency.html), it is tempting to use steroid-type sprays, the primary effect of which is cooling but drains yang without properly supplementing yin.

- where bacterial infection is suspected, antibiotics may be prescribed. These have a cold-damp effect. They usually kill the bug (assuming the antibiotic is well-chosen and the bacteria hasn't learned to resist it, now becoming a huge problem see http://www.theguardian.com/society/2014/may/22/antibiotic-resistant-bugs-health-drug) but, being cold and damp, can weaken the Spleen. That means that the phlegm remains and may increase.

As you see, although not deeply complicated, there are many ways in which phlegm can compromise the body. Making the right diagnosis and then treatment is not always easy.

For example, if the cause has been, say Heat invasion, but there is also an underlying Yin deficiency with Kidney Yang exhaustion (as can happen with the elderly) and a history of bad diet, picking one's way through the treatment process can take time – and perseverance from the patient.

Here the weak Kidney Yang cannot transform fluids, which then overflow upwards and stagnate. Guess what happens? Those fluids, under the drying/heating effect of Yin deficiency and bad diet, (most of which is heating in effect), then transform back into phlegm!

If you have phlegm that you cannot diagnose as being from fatigue, damp, cold, heat or dryness, you need to see a specialist who understands phlegm. For Chinese medicine in the British Isles go to https://www.acupuncture.org.uk.

## Your Review?

*Finally ...*

Now you've read this book, *please review it!* As implied in the introduction, it aims to be not just informative, but *useful*.

If you think others would benefit from it, please post your opinion somewhere prospective readers might see it, such as on Amazon.

Here are links to the North American site (https://www.amazon.com) and the UK site (https://www.amazon.co.uk).

- Just click on the link above (either amazon.com or amazon.co.uk – or of course, your own country's equivalent)

- Put "Yuck! Phlegm!" in the search box at the top of the Amazon page

- When a picture of the book appears, click on where it says 'review' or 'reviews', then

- Click on "Write a customer review" and say what you think about it:

- You can give it 5 stars out of 5 – if you think it merits them, of course!

I hope you will be positive and constructive, but if you have major criticisms or reservations, I would like to know! Then I can improve it for the next person.

You can also let me know through my website http://www.acupuncture-points.org on many pages of which there is a box for writing to me.

# Appendix - Preparing Herbs

## PREPARING HERBS

### Decoction

For most plants where the parts used are hard or fibrous, such as twigs, roots, barks, decocting is the traditional way to extract beneficial qualities.

First slice or crush the parts of the plant to be used; place them in a pan made of glass, porcelain, enamel or earthenware – preferably no metal should be in contact with the plant. Cover with enough cold water that, once brought to boil, covered and very gently simmered for up to 30 minutes, will leave about 450 millilitres. About 30g of the plant is enough for 600 mls to start with, which after simmering reduces to 450mls.

After cooling, strain the mixture, discarding the plant. Divide the liquid into three parts of 150ml each. Keep these in the refridgerator. Drink 150mls , unsweetened, but with a little warm water added, about 30 minutes before each of the main three meals in a day.

### Short Decoction

Short decoctions are used where the parts of the plant are less fibrous, for example for leaves, seeds and fruits. The difference is that the plant is simmered only for about 10 minutes, then allowed to remain in the cooling liquid for another 10 minutes ('steeping' it.)

First cut or crush the parts of the plant to be used; place them in a pan made of glass, porcelain, enamel or earthenware – preferably no metal should be in contact with the plant. Cover with enough cold water that, once brought to boil, covered and very gently simmered for up to 10 minutes, will leave about 450 millilitres. (Usually about 30g of the plant is enough for 500 mls to start with, which after simmering for 10 minutes reduces to 450mls.)

After cooling, strain the mixture, discarding the plant. Divide the liquid into three parts of 150ml each. Keep these in the refrigerator. Drink 150mls , unsweetened, but with a little warm water added, about 30 minutes before each of the main three meals in a day.

## Infusion

This method is used where the parts of the plant are lighter and much less fibrous, and may have been dried, such as stems, flowers and leaves.

Place 500ml water in an enamel, glass, earthenware or porcelain pan. Bring it to the boil and pour in 30gm of the plant: immediately turn off the source of heat and cover the pan with a well-fitting cap or lid. Leave it to cool and infuse for about 20 minutes.

Strain the liquid, and divide into three parts. Refrigerate them. Drink one part about 30 minutes before a meal, having added warm water to it beforehand, three times daily.

## Sun Tea infusion

This is used where the aromatic or essential oils in the plant play an important part in how it works.

Instead of using boiling water, cold water is placed in a glass jar with the herbs and left in the sun all day – preferably for at least 6-8 hours. After straining, the liquid is again refrigerated. One third of it is consumed on an empty stomach three times daily, with a little warm water added to each dose beforehand.

## Syrup

Syrups are made with lots of sugar, honey, molasses or other sweetener, which has a soothing and yin enhancing benefit on inflamed tissues.

Taken for too long, syrups – not matter how beneficial the herbs they contain – will eventually weaken your Spleen function, leading to phlegm formation. You have been warned!

First, make your syrup. Add 1 lb (450gms) sugar (or other sweetener) to 1 pint (500 mls) of hot water in an enamel, earthenware, glass or porcelain pot over heat. Stir until all the sugar has dissolved, then remove from heat and continue to stir until it is cool. Pour into clean bottles for safe-keeping.

There are various ways of combining the syrup with the herbs. The following is the simplest.

Take 500 mls and add to 500 mls of the herbal decoction. Heat until boiling, stirring throughout, then remove from the heat and continue to stir as it cools. Keep in well covered jars or bottles.

## Essential oils

These you must buy as preparing them requires careful manufacturing quality control.

http://www.snowlotus.org/about-snow-lotus-essential-oils

# Bibliography - select

## GENERAL BOOKS, EASY TO READ

### For lung efficiency

The Oxygen Advantage – Patrick McKeown – pub William Morrow & Company

Breathe: The Simple, Revolutionary 14-Day Program to Improve Your Mental and Physical Health – Belisa Vranich – pub St. Martin's Griffin

### Stress seen from Chinese medicine's perspective

Qi Stagnation – Signs of Stress – Jonathan Clogstoun-Willmott – pub Frame of Mind Publishing

### If you are often low-spirited or cold

Yang Deficiency – Get your Fire Burning Again! – Jonathan Clogstoun-Willmott – pub Frame of Mind Publishing

## If you suffer from Dry Phlegm, or are exhausted or burnt-out

Yin Deficiency – Burnout and Exhaustion, What to Do! – Jonathan
   Clogstoun-Willmott – pub Frame of Mind Publishing

## A well-known book about food

Chinese System of Food Cures – Henry Lu – pub Sterling


## BOOKS FOR PROFESSIONALS, NEEDING TECHNICAL KNOWLEDGE/UNDERSTANDING

Aging and Blood Stasis – Yan De-Xin – pub Poppy Press
Blood Stasis – Gunter Neeb –  pub Churchill Livingstone
Chinese Herbal Medicine Formulas and Strategies – Bensky & Barolet –
   pub Eastland Press
Chinese Materia Medica – Bensky and Gamble – pub Eastfield Press
Fluid Physiology and Pathology in Traditional Chinese Medicine –
   Steven Clavey – pub Churchill Livingstone
Foundations of Chinese Medicine – Giovanni Macioca – pub Churchill
   Livingstone
Out of the Earth – Simon Mills – pub Viking
Prescription for Nutritional Healing – Balch and Balch – pub Avery
The Energetics of Western Herbs – Peter Holmes – pub Artemis
   available from http://www.snowlotus.org/books/

# About the Author

Jonathan Clogstoun-Willmott was raised on a farm in England, where he learned to appreciate the joys of milk and phlegm.

Later, he got a degree in Electrical Engineering, a mistake.

He followed that by qualifying as a Chartered Accountant, a worse mistake.

Then he got ill, the best thing that happened because he met someone who cured and mentored him.

So he took up Chinese medicine. Since 1977 he has practised various forms of alternative medicine, all based round or explicable in Chinese medicine.

He moved to Edinburgh, Scotland in 1982.

He has two adult children and a wonderful wife.

He likes the hypnogogic state you enter as you go to sleep, preferably accompanied by a Mozart piano concerto.

He sees patients. He gardens. He lectures. He plays the piano badly so as to distract himself.

He writes a website (http://www.acupuncture-points.org) and occasional books.

'Yuck! Phlegm!' is his fourth book that uses Chinese medicine to explain health and life.